CHOOSING FOODS
for a
HEALTHY HEART

CHOOSING
FOODS
for a
HEALTHY
HEART

Michael Mogadam, M.D.

CONSUMER REPORTS BOOKS
A DIVISION OF CONSUMERS UNION
YONKERS, NEW YORK

Copyright © 1993 by Michael Mogadam

Published by Consumers Union of United States, Inc., Yonkers, New York 10703.

LIBRARY OF CONGRESS CATALOGING-IN-PUBLICATION DATA
Mogadam, Michael.
    Choosing foods for a healthy heart / by Michael Mogadam.
        p.   cm.
    Includes bibliographical references and index.
    ISBN 0-89043-633-9
    1. Coronary heart disease—Prevention.   2. Coronary heart disease—
Nutritional aspects.   I. Title.
    RC685.C6M65   1993
    616.1'2305—dc20   92-39213
                                                                  CIP

This book was printed on recycled paper.

Design by Kathryn Parise

First printing, June 1993

Manufactured in the United States of America

Choosing Foods for a Healthy Heart is a Consumer Reports Book published by Consumers Union, the nonprofit organization that publishes *Consumer Reports,* the monthly magazine of test reports, product Ratings, and buying guidance. Established in 1936, Consumers Union is chartered under the Not-For-Profit Corporation Law of the State of New York.

The purposes of Consumers Union, as stated in its charter, are to provide consumers with information and counsel on consumer goods and services, to give information on all matters relating to the expenditure of the family income, and to initiate and to cooperate with individual and group efforts seeking to create and maintain decent living standards.

Consumers Union derives its income solely from the sale of *Consumer Reports* and other publications. In addition, expenses of occasional public service efforts may be met, in part, by nonrestrictive, noncommercial contributions, grants, and fees. Consumers Union accepts no advertising or product samples and is not beholden in any way to any commercial interest. Its Ratings and reports are solely for the use of the readers of its publications. Neither the Ratings, nor the reports, nor any Consumers Union publication, including this book, may be used in advertising or for any commercial purpose. Consumers Union will take all steps open to it to prevent such uses of its material, its name, or the name of *Consumer Reports.*

*"Whether my observations and opinions
be disproved or supported, I shall be satisfied.
Truth is the prize aimed for; and in the contest,
there is at least this consolation that
all the competitors may share
equally the good attained."*

Sir Dominic John Corrigan
Lancet 1(1829): 586–90

Contents

Foreword

Coronary heart disease is the leading cause of mortality in the United States. Although there are numerous risk factors for coronary heart disease, nutritional and life-style practices can modify many of them. As a result, a program that presents clear, easy-to-follow guidelines to improve cardiovascular health can be an important asset in decreasing the risk of heart attack. Consumers Union's medical consultants believe that the CEF (Cardiovascular Effects of Food) Index is such a program.

The CEF Index, developed by Michael Mogadam, M.D., author of this book, provides a single summary number for each of several hundred common foods and prepared dishes. That number represents the combined effects—both positive and negative—of the nutrients in each food on the heart. According to Dr. Mogadam, if you keep your total CEF Index of all foods each day to no more than +30, you will probably be eating healthy foods for a healthy heart.

Although Dr. Mogadam's rationale for the CEF Index of foods embodies some accepted standards for heart-healthy eating, he also draws on a number of studies that are considered inconclusive or controversial by some practicing cardiologists and nutritionists. However, Consumers Union's consultants find the CEF Index to be sufficiently useful to justify publication of this book. We believe you'll find the CEF Index equally useful in choosing foods for a healthy heart.

THE EDITORS OF CONSUMER REPORTS BOOKS

Acknowledgment

Without the unceasing encouragement and dedication of Mrs. Ann Marie Galus, and her cheerful technical support for my endless revisions, the completion of this book would have been a far more difficult challenge. I will remain deeply grateful to her.

CHOOSING
FOODS
for a
HEALTHY
HEART

Introduction

❧

In the United States, cardiovascular diseases constitute a major public health problem: More than 69 million Americans have various cardiovascular disorders, including high blood pressure, coronary heart disease, and stroke. Each year 1.5 million people will have a heart attack, some while only in their thirties and forties. More Americans die of heart disease than from cancer, accidents, pneumonia, influenza, suicide, and AIDS combined. In 1992, heart and blood vessel diseases cost approximately $110 billion in medical services and lost productivity.

Personal responsibility for changes in life-styles and dietary practices is a major national goal for government and volunteer health agencies in the 1990s. Education for personal responsibility is the cornerstone of various public campaigns for health and medical interventions to reduce cardiovascular diseases and disabilities. The public is inundated with confusing, faddish, conflicting, and frequently inaccurate information about how and why various nutrients affect the cardiovascular system. *Choosing Foods for a Healthy Heart* provides the most recent in-depth explanation of cardiovascular effects of foods, while correcting many popular misconceptions. It also introduces a novel approach to nutrition for cardiovascular health.

Although there are more than 270 risk factors under consideration for coronary heart disease, in the past 40 years the nutritional approach to cardiovascular health has centered around high blood cholesterol and avoidance of dietary cholesterol and fat, particularly saturated fat. However, no food's health effects can be judged solely on the basis of cholesterol and fat content, because this narrow focus ignores the exceedingly diverse or even competing roles of different nutrients.

Choosing Foods for a Healthy Heart is the product of four years of extensive research that led to the creation of the CEF (*C*ardiovascular *E*ffects of *F*oods) Index. The CEF Index of a given food is a single number that represents the overall cardiovascular impact of all major nutrients in that food. These nutrients include dietary cholesterol, saturated fat, monounsaturated fat, different types of polyunsaturated fats, salt, dietary fiber, proteins, carbohydrates, vitamins, and minerals. Thus, the CEF Index is a comprehensive and far more meaningful gauge of the nutritional worth of the foods we eat than the current practice of focusing only on cholesterol or saturated fat. The CEF Index provides at a glance, and instantly, the total cardiovascular impact of a given food.

Choosing Foods for a Healthy Heart offers a practical and flexible dietary concept that allows you the freedom to choose your own foods at home or away from home without any rigid diet plan. The total CEF Index makes choosing your meals easy. It also avoids information overload and the confusion over how much of what ingredients are present in a given food and what these ingredients mean individually or when mixed with other ingredients.

The CEF indexes of nearly 1,000 common foods are provided to make food selection an enjoyable personal choice. A simple guide allows the consumer to easily figure out an approximate CEF index for any food not listed in the book.

Enjoy your reading, and share your knowledge.

1

Understanding Cholesterol

According to the World Health Organization, cardiovascular diseases are currently the number one public health problem worldwide. In this country, efforts to educate the public and health providers regarding the prevention and control of coronary heart disease have intensified since 1985, when the National Cholesterol Education Program (NCEP) was created. The NCEP, the American Heart Association (AHA), and the United States Public Health authorities consider an elevated blood cholesterol level to be a major risk factor for various cardiovascular events. For this reason, a nationwide campaign has been mounted to influence the public to alter their eating habits in order to reduce blood cholesterol levels.

To understand the concern and the controversy over blood cholesterol levels, the statistics summarized in Table 1.1 illustrate the magnitude of the problem.

The "Misunderstood" Cholesterol

Cholesterol is a pearly, fatlike substance present in all animal flesh and products but *not* in plants. It is so important to humans and animals that they could not live without it.

Only 7 percent of the total body cholesterol in humans actually

TABLE 1.1

**Estimated Prevalence of Elevated Blood Cholesterol Levels
in the United States**

Population Size	Cholesterol Levels* (mg/dl)
100 million	>200
70 percent of individuals 45 to 74 years of age	>200
33 percent of men and 50 percent of women	>240
47 million	>240
24 million individuals over 55 years of age	>240
25 percent of all adults	>240

(mg/dl = milligrams per deciliter; > = greater than)

*Values of 200–239 mg/dl are considered "borderline high," and those greater than 240 are "high."

circulates in the blood. The remaining 93 percent is scattered throughout the body in various organs. A substantial part of circulating blood cholesterol is taken up by the liver and converted to bile, which then flows into the upper intestine. Bile is essential for the digestion and absorption of various fats and fat-soluble vitamins. Cholesterol is also used by the gonads to produce sex hormones and by the adrenal glands to produce vital steroidlike hormones.

It is now generally agreed that for those under the age of 60, a total blood cholesterol level under 200 mg/dl is "desirable," 200 to 239 mg/dl is "borderline high," and 240 mg/dl or above is "high." Since nearly all biological values change with aging, one must add 10 mg/dl for each five years of life past the age of 60 (see Table 1.2). For example, in a 70-year-old person, a total blood cholesterol level of 220 mg/dl is considered acceptable.

TABLE 1.2

Age-Adjusted Total Blood Cholesterol (and LDL) Levels*

	Age to 60	*Age 65*	*Age 70*	*Age 75*
Desirable	<200	<210	<220	<230
	(<130)	(<135)	(<140)	(<145)
Borderline	200–240	210–250	220–260	230–270
	(130–160)	(135–165)	(140–170)	(145–175)
High	>240	>250	>260	>270
	(>160)	(>165)	(>170)	(>175)

< = Less than

> = Greater than

LDL = low-density lipoprotein cholesterol

*All levels shown are mg/dl. A 10-mg/dl increment is allowed for total cholesterol for each five years past the age of 60. The increment for LDL cholesterol is 5 mg/dl. For HDL cholesterol, any value *below* 45 mg/dl for men and *below* 55 mg/dl for women is considered undesirable.

The Sources of Blood Cholesterol

There is a common misconception that dietary cholesterol is the only source of blood cholesterol. But circulating blood cholesterol actually comes from the food we eat *and* from cholesterol produced in our bodies, especially in the intestines and the liver. Even if we follow a cholesterol-free diet, the liver will continue to convert other foods into cholesterol, as it does in all animals. Cattle, for example, eat no cholesterol, get very little saturated fat from their feed, and have a diet that is rich in complex carbohydrates. Yet cattle produce lots of fat (a substantial portion of it saturated) and plenty of cholesterol (in both meat and dairy products). Cattle therefore represent efficient factories for taking in "desirable" nutrients and making a number of "undesirable" products. Chickens also eat no cholesterol and an insignificant amount of saturated fat, but they lay eggs that contain on average about 220 mg of cholesterol each.

Cholesterol "Responders"

It is estimated that in only 30 percent of humans do blood cholesterol levels change in response to dietary cholesterol intake. Such persons can be called cholesterol "responders." In other words, even when most people restrict their intake of dietary cholesterol, the change in total blood cholesterol levels will usually be less than 10 percent. Studies around the world have consistently shown that even a moderate cholesterol intake (such as a diet containing several eggs per week) fails to raise blood cholesterol levels in approximately 70 percent of the population, who are cholesterol "nonresponders" (see chapter 6). In fact, dietary cholesterol is far less important than saturated fat in changing the level and the composition of blood cholesterol, or in increasing the risk of cardiovascular events.

Lipoproteins:
The "Good," the "Bad," and the "Mean"

In circulating blood, oxygen is carried by red blood cells to various tissues. Many substances in the blood, including cholesterol, must be transported by some other means in order to get around. Nature's "vehicles" for transporting cholesterol throughout the body are lipoproteins (a mixture of lipids and proteins). Lipoproteins look like tiny golf balls. Inside they are packed with cholesterol and various fats called triglycerides; their thin outer cobblestone-like shell contains cholesterol, complex fats, and proteins in an ever-changing mix. So what we refer to as "blood cholesterol" is carried by these particles of various lipoproteins, which are different from and more complex than dietary cholesterol alone.

Lipoproteins are usually classified on the basis of their density or compactness. The more protein (and the less fat) they contain, the more compact (or dense) they are. Although their names may sound intimidating, they aren't that hard to remember. Four of the five important lipoproteins are recognized by their density:

FIGURE 1.1

Structure of High-Density Lipoprotein Particles

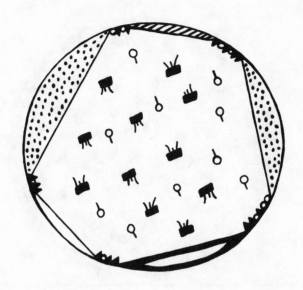

⬭ Apoprotein A-1		O Cholesterol	
⬤ Apoprotein A-2		▲ Complex fats	
⬤ Apoprotein C		♀ Cholesterol bound to a fatty acid	
⬤ Apoprotein E		♈ Triglycerides	

very-low-density lipoproteins (VLDL), intermediate-density lipoproteins (IDL), low-density lipoproteins (LDL), and high-density
lipoproteins (HDL). The fifth lipoprotein, which is highly damaging to the inner wall of coronary arteries, is lipoprotein (a), or
Lp(a) (pronounced "LP little a"). All lipoproteins except HDL
transport cholesterol throughout the body and sometimes deposit
it in the walls of coronary arteries. For this "heart-unfriendly"
behavior, cholesterol carried by the lower-density varieties

FIGURE 1.2

Structure of
Low-Density Lipoprotein Particles

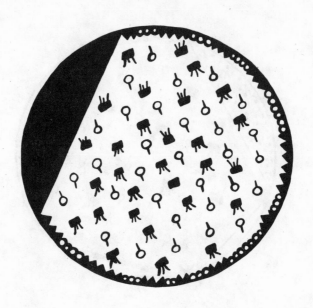

⏴ Apoprotein B

O Cholesterol

▲ Complex fats

♀ Cholesterol bound to
a fatty acid

🎋 Triglycerides

(VLDL, IDL, and LDL) is known as the "bad" cholesterol. HDL, on the other hand, carries the excess cholesterol away from the arteries, creating a "reverse transport." For this reason, its cholesterol is called, appropriately, the "good" cholesterol.

LDL has two close relatives that are even more damaging to coronary arteries. Because of this mean behavior, we can call their cholesterol the "mean" cholesterol. One kind is produced when LDL is oxidized (becomes rancid). Oxidized LDL is more easily picked up by certain white blood cells (monocytes), which may creep into the walls of coronary arteries, where they accumulate over time. This is the beginning of a fatty "streak" that can eventually turn into hardened plaque.

Small amounts of LDL's other relative, Lp(a), are present along with other lipoproteins in everyone. It is only when the blood level of Lp(a) goes above 25 to 30 mg/dl that it may become a major risk factor for coronary artery disease. In fact, for many African-Americans with coronary heart disease, and for Caucasian men under 60 with high total cholesterol levels, LP(a) may be a far more important contributing factor than "bad" LDL cholesterol. In addition to cholesterol accumulation in the arteries, Lp(a) may also contribute to blood clots, which is often the final straw that causes a heart attack.

Like automobiles, lipoproteins come in different types, or subclasses. For examples, one subclass of LDL (LDL-3) can cause severe damage to coronary arteries, whereas another subclass (LDL-1) is unlikely to have any major adverse effects on the heart. The third type (LDL-2) is a straddler: It can convert to either the harmful or the neutral LDL. The cardiovascular benefit of the "good" HDL is mostly provided by the HDL-2 subclass, and to a lesser degree by HDL-3 (there are five kinds of HDL).

The existence of these subclasses may explain, in part, why many individuals with abnormal blood cholesterol levels do not develop coronary heart disease. For example, just because the LDL cholesterol is up does not mean that the unfriendly LDL-3 subclass is the culprit. For the same reason, the protection afforded by the "good" HDL against "bad" cholesterol cannot be accurately estimated without knowing their various subclasses. A useful tool is the ratio of total cholesterol (TC) to HDL cholesterol (HDL-C), which can be calculated by dividing TC by HDL-C. A ratio under 4 is considered desirable by many experts.

Apoproteins: The Agents of Lipoproteins

All lipoproteins, as the vehicles for cholesterol, have substances that determine where they go and what happens to their cholesterol. These agents, the protein elements of lipoproteins, are called apoproteins (or apo). They are the most important substances in the entire lipoprotein system because they determine what kind of lipoprotein is formed. They control the behavior of the "good," "bad," and "mean" cholesterols. The most important apoproteins are the cardioprotective apo A-1 (which belongs to HDL cholesterol) and the coronary unfriendly apo B-100 (which belongs to LDL cholesterol).

Variability of Test Results

Knowing your total blood cholesterol is a good first step toward cardiovascular health. But simply knowing the total blood cholesterol level is not enough—you also need to find out the levels of cholesterol carried by the "good" and "bad" lipoproteins as well as the level of triglycerides. Measuring total blood cholesterol counts the cholesterol carried by all the vehicles (lipoproteins) traveling on a highway (the blood vessel). These vehicles come in different shapes and sizes and transport different cargo (various fats, cholesterol, and proteins); some carry cholesterol to the cells, and some take it away. More important, their mix changes almost continuously.

A major source of error in recording blood cholesterol levels is that such levels can vary from day to day and from week to week. (This is also true for a wide range of other blood tests.) Many factors can change the results of blood cholesterol analysis:

- Nonstandardized laboratories. Finger sticks and cholesterol screenings at shopping malls should not be accepted as the last word. If you get a reading that is over 200 mg/dl, have your doctor recheck it.
- Smoking before a blood test, which may give higher values
- Not fasting for 12 or more hours before the test. A meal will change the lipoprotein analysis, especially the triglyceride level.
- Different body positions. Cholesterol levels tend to be

higher if we sit up while blood is being drawn; levels are lower when we lie flat.

- Applying the tourniquet for more than two or three minutes may give a 5 to 7 percent higher value.
- Time of day (Morning levels are lower.)
- Time of year (Winter levels are usually higher.)
- Exercise, dieting, a change in body weight, phase of a woman's menstrual cycle, or taking estrogen/ progesterone and certain other medications (The values may vary.)
- Various acute and chronic illnesses (Usually the values are lower.)

Even when all of the above factors are carefully controlled, cholesterol levels still can fluctuate by as much as 20 percent from week to week.

If a random test for blood cholesterol is under 200 mg/dl, most adults without a family history of cardiovascular disease do not require additional testing. However, those with higher levels need two or three lipoprotein analyses (not just the total cholesterol level) after 12 to 14 hours of fasting. These analyses should be done at least several weeks apart.

Lipoprotein analysis is a readily available test. When performed properly, it provides valuable information. Among various pieces of information within a lipoprotein analysis, some experts believe that VLDL and HDL cholesterol levels and the ratio of total cholesterol to HDL cholesterol are better indicators of the risk for coronary heart disease than the LDL level alone.

We use abbreviations such as LDL, HDL, etc., when discussing lipoprotein analysis, but what is measured is cholesterol content; the test gives us no information about the rest of the lipoprotein components. Additional testing for some of these components, such as the blood levels of apo A-1 and B-100 (associated with the "good" HDL and the "bad" LDL, respectively), and lipoprotein (a) are at times extremely valuable. When there is a personal or family history of coronary heart disease at a young age, or when someone with coronary heart disease has a lipoprotein-cholesterol analysis within the desirable range, these special tests may reveal other important lipid abnormalities.

Lipoprotein Analysis

A lipoprotein analysis should *always* include the following:

Blood Lipids	*Desirable Range*
Total cholesterol	<200 mg/dl
High-density lipoprotein (HDL)	>45 mg/dl
Low-density lipoprotein (LDL)	<130 mg/dl
Very-low-density lipoprotein (VLDL)	<30 mg/dl
Triglycerides	<120 mg/dl
Cholesterol/HDL ratio	<4

< = less than
> = greater than

Note: Intermediate-density lipoprotein is usually measured along with the VLDL.

2

The ABCs of
Coronary Heart Disease

❦

Coronary heart disease (CHD), unlike strep throat or a broken bone, does not have a readily identifiable cause. For decades health professionals, agencies, and organizations have told the public that dietary fat, cholesterol, and salt are the culprits. But coronary heart disease is almost always a multifactorial disease, with several factors participating at various times to injure the arteries or sustain them.

So far, more than 270 risk factors, but not causes, for CHD have been identified. Every risk factor increases the likelihood (or the risk) that a particular disease or event may occur. When multiple risk factors coexist, invariably the potential for disease and its associated complications is increased. However, it is impossible to accurately quantify or estimate the relative importance of many CHD risk factors, because a given risk (or risks) may be relevant to one individual and not present at all in others. For example, if a car's windshield wipers break while someone is driving in rain or snow, this is a definite risk factor for a traffic accident. But so are bad brakes, icy roads, driving while intoxicated, and other factors. Whereas one or more of these risk factors may be relevant to a given accident, most or all may be absent in a large number of other accidents.

Given the limitations of ranking various coronary heart disease

TABLE 2.1

Major Risk Factors for Coronary Heart Disease (CHD)

1. Personal history of cardiovascular events

2. Family history of CHD, especially at a young age

3. Age: People over 45 are at higher risk.

4. Smoking

5. Low blood HDL-cholesterol

6. Diabetes

7. Inappropriate response or resistance to insulin (particularly in overweight or obese persons)

8. Gender: Men and postmenopausal women are at risk.

9. Elevated blood LDL-cholesterol (LDL-3 subclass)

10. Abnormal blood levels of various other lipids

11. An enlarged heart, usually from high blood pressure or obesity

12. Hypertension

13. Abdominal obesity

14. Abnormal blood platelets

15. An elevated blood level of homocysteine (a genetic disorder)

16. High levels of various clotting factors in the blood, especially fibrinogen

17. Excess iron in the body

18. Bacterial or viral injury of the arterial wall (by herpes, cytomegaloviruses, etc.)

19. High intake of saturated and trans fatty acids

20. Low level of physical fitness—sedentary life-style

risk factors, the important ones are listed in Table 2.1. Although the order of ranking may be applicable to a large population, it will vary from individual to individual.

Emotional disorders such as dissatisfaction with work, family, or life; overwhelming responsibility; marital conflict; or losing a spouse through death or divorce are minor risk factors. Recent studies suggest, however, that many emotional and psychiatric disorders are associated with abnormal levels of adrenaline-like chemicals in the blood called catecholamines, which lower the "good" HDL-cholesterol level and may also provoke clot formation within the coronary arteries. Thus, the apparent increased risk of coronary heart disease in many emotional disorders may be related to the biochemical abnormalities found among the major risk factors.

Coronary heart disease is usually brought on by multiple risk factors over many years. Many important risk factors are genetic. Nevertheless, no matter what genes we inherit from our parents, how or when they show up can be changed significantly by altering our own life-styles.

The Process of Coronary Heart Disease

Coronary arteries, very much like thin-walled rubber tubes, are elastic; they can stretch and then go back to their original size in response to the heart's contractions and the flow of blood. However, many risk factors can change this elasticity, resulting in the stiffening or hardening of the arteries.

Hardening of the arteries may begin with some injury to the very thin inner wall of the arteries—the endothelium. Initially, if the damage is minor, it does not provoke a significant amount of inflammation or thickening of the wall. However, if the damage is deeper and disrupts the endothelium, causing chapping and sores, then a more vigorous response occurs. For example, LDL and Lp(a) particles, along with certain white blood cells (called monocytes), go through these cracks into the arterial wall. There the LDL and Lp(a) particles are oxidized and promptly gobbled up by monocytes, creating "foamy" cells in the arterial wall. When these "foamy" cells eventually burst, a lot of scarring and inflammation follows, resulting in an uneven and hardened plaque or bulge, called an atheroma. When there are many atheromas, the condition is then referred to as hardening (sclerosis) of the arteries, or atherosclerosis.

Hardening of the arteries is a slow and usually progressive process that can take 20 to 30 years to become apparent or cause symptoms. Millions of people, especially older persons, can continue for years living normal lives in spite of some atherosclerosis. But when the accumulated plaque narrows the artery to a critical point (which varies for each person), the amount of blood flow and oxygen to the heart muscle may be inadequate, especially during times of exertion or stress. This relative oxygen deficiency, called ischemia, usually causes heart pain (angina). But some people have silent ischemia—that is, ischemia without pain.

For a heart attack to occur, something else has to happen to an atherosclerotic artery. The culprits here are blood platelets that stick to these eroded plaques, trapping red and white blood cells to form a clot (thrombosis). As the clot becomes larger and larger, it may nearly or totally block the artery, causing coronary thrombosis or myocardial infarction—heart attack.

Atherosclerosis in its early stages is very much reversible. However, once the plaques have established themselves (similar to water pipes clogged by years of hardened sediment), the best we can hope for is to alleviate the symptoms or reduce the risk of having a heart attack or stroke. We can never make the arteries normal again.

3

The Impact of Abnormal
Blood Cholesterol
Levels

In the United States, over 6 million persons—about 2 percent of
the entire population—have been diagnosed with coronary heart
disease (CHD). Another 3 million have had strokes. There are also
approximately 60 million Americans with high blood pressure. Of
course, millions of older adults may have hardening of the arteries
to various degrees, although it may not cause any symptoms and
can go undiagnosed. For most people, changes in coronary arteries are slight and will not cause any problems. The same can be said
of minor arthritis, which affects many older persons but doesn't
have an important effect on their life expectancy or quality of life.

After menopause, a far greater number of women have elevated
blood cholesterol levels than do men. This higher average blood
cholesterol level results in a greater risk of coronary heart disease
for postmenopausal women. Even so, women generally have a
lower rate of CHD than do men of the same age, but the gap closes
after the age of 60.

Overall, only 1 percent of men and women age 30 to 39 and
only 10 percent of those between 60 and 69 have coronary heart
disease. Although the sheer number of Americans who have CHD
is huge (6 million), most of the 100 million with elevated blood

cholesterol levels will not develop CHD. Obviously, coronary heart disease is the result of a complex process and multiple risk factors, but more research is needed before we can predict which persons with elevated cholesterol will develop this disease.

The Significance of Elevated Blood Cholesterol

Approximately one-fourth (or about 1.5 million) of Americans with CHD have elevated levels of blood cholesterol. In other words, of the estimated 75 to 100 million Americans with "high" or "borderline high" blood cholesterol, only 1.5 percent now have coronary heart disease. Millions are still in the incubation period, which can last 20 to 30 years. For a large number of people, the problem is not just an isolated elevation of the "bad" LDL cholesterol, since they often have other lipid abnormalities, especially high levels of the "mean" lipoprotein (a) or low levels of the "good" HDL cholesterol. Many recent studies of persons with documented coronary heart disease show that, in 70 to 80 percent of cases, the problem is not elevated blood levels of the "bad" LDL cholesterol but rather low levels of the "good" HDL cholesterol.

Clearly, most people with elevated levels of blood cholesterol do not develop symptomatic coronary heart disease. The reverse is also true: Most people with CHD do not have elevated blood cholesterol levels, but they often have other blood lipid abnormalities. Even though a slight-to-moderate elevation of blood cholesterol (200 to 239 mg/dl), in the absence of other important risk factors, does not significantly increase the risk of CHD, the presence of *other* risk factors—such as smoking coupled with high blood pressure—dramatically increases the risk of CHD. In addition, a history of heart attack alone will increase the risk of dying from another heart attack by 600 percent in those who already have "high" blood cholesterol (over 240 mg/dl). (See Table 3.1.)

Unfortunately, multiple risk factors are common, and they fre-

TABLE 3.1

**Death Rates from Coronary Heart Disease
Based on Multiple Risk Factors***

Blood Cholesterol (mg/dl)	Nonsmokers with Normal Blood Pressure	Smokers with High Blood Pressure
Under 181	1.6	6.3
182–202	2.5	10.
203–221	2.7	15.5
222–245	3.8	16.6
Over 245	6.4	21.4

*Middle-aged and older men (per 1,000 annually)

quently result in an even greater risk of death from various cardiovascular diseases.

The Significance of Low "Good" HDL Cholesterol

The fact that only 20 to 30 percent of persons with CHD have elevated blood cholesterol does not mean that the other 70 to 80 percent have no other abnormalities in their blood lipids. What can be said with certainty is that in many persons with CHD, the other risk factors listed in Table 2.1 are just as important as the blood levels of the "bad" LDL.

Abnormal levels of other lipoproteins or apoproteins contribute heavily to coronary heart disease. In fact, nearly all recent studies have consistently shown that in both men and women, the blood level of the "bad" LDL cholesterol is far less important than the blood level of the "good" HDL cholesterol.

In women, HDL cholesterol levels are about 25 percent higher than they are in men of the same age—a difference that, in part, accounts for lower rates of CHD in women. And 80 percent of women with documented coronary heart disease have undesirably low HDL cholesterol levels—below 45 mg/dl.

The "good" HDL cholesterol is thought to prevent atherosclerosis by carrying cholesterol from the arterial wall to the liver for processing. The HDL also reduces the oxidation of the "bad" LDL and its conversion into the "mean" LDL.

It is estimated that for every 1-mg/dl increase in the "good" HDL, there is a 4 percent *decrease* in the risk of coronary heart disease, whereas for every 1-mg/dl increase in the "bad" LDL, the risk of cardiovascular events increases by 2 percent.

The Significance of Elevated Triglycerides and the "Bad" VLDL Cholesterol

Edible fats are absorbed by the intestine in the form of triglycerides (a glycerin molecule holding three fatty acids), then carried by tiny fat particles called chylomicrons (pronounced kyle-o-MIKE-rons). The blood carries these particles to muscles, fat cells, and other tissues where, within 15 to 30 minutes, some of their fatty acids are stripped away for use by these tissues or for storage in fat cells. The remnants of these chylomicrons are then taken up by the liver, which removes even more of the components, and are returned to the blood as the "bad" VLDL. This VLDL still contains 50 to 65 percent triglycerides. After some "remodeling," VLDL is eventually cleared from the blood by the liver and other tissues.

So long as this orderly process is not interrupted, the blood levels of triglycerides and VLDL remain stable. However, there are a host of genetic or acquired disorders in which this orderly process is interrupted somewhere along the line, resulting in accumulation of the "bad" VLDL and triglycerides in the blood circulation. Almost always, elevated triglycerides make a bad situation even worse by lowering the blood level of the "good" HDL. Consequently, the negative cardiovascular impact of elevated triglycerides is far greater than an isolated elevation of the "bad" LDL cholesterol. A recent study from Germany (the PROCAM Study) of 4,559 men 40 to 65 years of age showed that elevated triglycerides, when accompanied by low HDL and high LDL levels, increased the risk of heart attacks tenfold!

It is important to emphasize that for too long we have focused on elevated levels of blood cholesterol, not realizing that in nearly 3 out of 4 persons with coronary heart disease, the culprit may be elevated triglycerides and VLDL, a low level of protective HDL, or a host of other lipid abnormalities. An isolated elevation of LDL is present in only 1 out of 4 persons with CHD. Recent studies have shown that in persons surviving an acute heart attack, the blood levels of triglycerides, apoprotein B, VLDL, and HDL (in that order) are more likely than LDL levels to be abnormal. In Japan, where elevated blood cholesterol is less common than in the United States, coronary heart disease is frequently associated with high blood levels of VLDL cholesterol and triglycerides, rather than with elevated LDL cholesterol.

4

Estimating the Risk
of a Future Heart Attack

❧

One major problem in dealing with risk factors rather than causes is the uncertainty regarding which people with abnormal blood lipids will develop coronary heart disease. Since the coexistence of several risk factors is known to increase the chances of CHD, obviously it is wise to reduce as many risk factors as possible.

Tables 4.1 and 4.2 provide a scoring system for estimating the cardiovascular impact of multiple risk factors. The scoring system is partially adapted from data available from the National Heart, Lung, and Blood Institute; the American Heart Association; and the Framingham Heart Study. But it is broadly modified to allow for the impact of the most common risk factors. To calculate your chances or probability of having coronary heart disease within the next 10 years, add all of the applicable scores (pluses *and* minuses) in Table 4.1. Then find the corresponding 10-year probability of experiencing a major coronary event in Table 4.2.

For example, if you are a 44-year-old male (+6), have high blood pressure (+5), smoke (+5), are 30 pounds overweight mostly around your waistline (+5), have a blood cholesterol level of 265 mg/dl (+4) and an HDL ("good") cholesterol level of 34 mg/dl (+7), and do not exercise regularly (+5), your total score is +37. Table 4.2 shows that your chance of having a coronary event in the next 10 years is greater than 50 percent. On the other hand, if you are a 44-year-old woman (+2) who does not have high blood pressure, obesity, abnormal blood lipids, or other

TABLE 4.1

Scoring System for Cardiovascular Risk Prevention

Age				Cholesterol (mg/dl)			
Female		**Male**		**Total**		**HDL**	
	Score		*Score*		*Score*		*Score*
Under 30	−10	Under 30	−2	Under 180	−1	Under 30	+10
30–34	−8	30–31	−1	180–199	0	30–35	+7
35–37	−5	32	0	200–239	+1	36–39	+4
38–39	−1	33–35	+1	240–269	+4	40–45	+3
40	0	36–40	+4	270–299	+6	46–49	0
41–44	+2	41–45	+6	Over 300	+8	50–55	−1
45–49	+4	46–49	+8			56–59	−3
50–59	+6	50–59	+10			60–69	−5
60–69	+8	60–69	+12			70–79	−7
Over 70	+10	Over 70	+14			Over 80	−10

Other Risk Factors	Score	*Other Protective Factors*	Score
Hypertension	+5	Daily dietary CEF Index below +30*	−5
Smoking	+5		
Diabetes	+5	Regular, vigorous exercise 3–4 times a week	−5
Elevated triglycerides	+5		
Abdominal obesity	+5	No family history of CHD	−5
Sedentary life-style	+5	Absence of *all* seven risk factors in left-hand column	−10
Family history of CHD before age 60	+10		
Personal history of CHD	+20		

*For CEF Index of foods, consult chapters 14–18.

TABLE 4.2

**Ten-Year Probability of a
Coronary Event**

Total Scores	Probability (percent)
1–5	2
6–8	5
9–12	6
13–16	10
17–19	15
20–23	20
24–25	25
26–28	30
29–30	35
31–35	40
Over 36	More than 50

major risk factors, you have practically no probability of experiencing a coronary event before your 54th birthday. Of course, these probabilities may go higher or lower depending on whether the other risk factors listed in Table 2.1 are present (see page 14).

You may wish to use the scoring system at this point to find out your risk level. Even if you do not have or know all the information (for example, your level of HDL cholesterol), use the scores for risk factors you know. If you come up with a high probability for a cardiovascular event, don't despair. The following chapters provide the necessary tools to reduce your risk or to keep it at the lowest possible level.

No matter what genetic or environmental factors are contributing to your risk of cardiovascular events, it helps to reduce all the risk factors you can. What is required is a "package" of dietary and nondietary changes rather than an isolated focus on a single risk factor.

5

Dietary Interventions for a Healthy Heart

❦

In the United States, cardiovascular diseases account for nearly 1 million, or 46 percent, of all deaths reported each year. Heart attack is the leading cause of death in the United States. Each year half a million people die from heart attacks, and 60 percent of these people die before they ever reach a hospital. For those dying from coronary heart disease (especially outside the hospital), all the sophisticated and expensive medical technology available is worthless. And unless preventive measures are adopted, people who are now 20, 30, or 40 years of age will experience a similar risk of cardiovascular events in the future.

The average life span in the United States has risen in this century from 47 to 76 years (79 for women, 74 for men). Dramatic reductions in infant and child mortality rates account for a substantial part of this increase in life expectancy. However, data from the United States Special Committee on Aging show that during the 1980s the population of Americans over 65 years of age grew 56 percent, and those over age 85 grew 65 percent. It is estimated that this trend will continue beyond the year 2020. If so, more people will live into their eighties and nineties. More important, this older population will include a large proportion of people suffering from hardening of the arteries as well as CHD complications. Preventive measures, including early intervention, might reduce the rate of various cardiovascular events or suffering, and the enormous cost of providing medical care for these individuals. This early intervention must be selective, practical, and flexible to allow long-term adherence to healthy dietary practices and life-styles.

The Limits of Short-term Dietary Intervention

Coronary artery disease does not happen overnight or even in a few weeks or years. Nor will it go away in a short time, no matter what we do. In fact, once coronary arteries develop plaques, they will never be normal again, in spite of changes in diet, medication, or even coronary artery bypass surgery. What is hoped for is to prevent the development of atherosclerosis in the first place, or to reduce the severity of the existing coronary artery disease and improve the blood flow to the heart muscle.

Dietary and life-style changes constitute the cornerstone of risk reduction. Although these changes may make you feel better after only a few weeks, the real benefits may require years to affect the heart's arteries. Short-term intervention studies (four to six years) to prevent cardiovascular events usually fail to show a significant benefit. On the other hand, many long-term studies (more than six years) confirm that reducing various risk factors through smoking cessation, adequate treatment of hypertension, lowering the level of "bad" LDL cholesterol, and raising the level of the "good" HDL cholesterol, or the modification of other major risk factors, will dramatically decrease various cardiovascular events. Since the benefits and rewards of short-term risk reduction do not last indefinitely, healthy life-styles that are practical over time should be adopted.

The Timing of Dietary Intervention

It stands to reason that reducing or eliminating risk factors at any age will cut down or prevent the likelihood of CHD. However, early intervention, before any significant damage has been done, is clearly more effective. Once atherosclerosis has set in, efforts such as dietary changes, reduction of various risk factors, or the use of drugs to correct cholesterol abnormalities may only modify the problem. However, stopping or reducing the progression of atherosclerosis is still possible.

Recommendations for Change

For millions of symptom-free and apparently healthy adults who are perfectly happy with what they eat, many issues must be considered before embarking on long-term dietary changes. These issues include the quality of life; personal tastes, habits, choices, and flexibility; cost; and the ease with which the diet can be followed at home and away from home (including at work). It should also be simple and understandable.

Most physicians have now abandoned rigid dietary programs such as no-salt diets (for kidney, liver, and heart diseases), sugar-free or low-carbohydrate diets (for diabetics), or bland and fat-free diets (for digestive or gallbladder disorders). It is equally unnecessary to insist on rigid dietary recommendations for millions of people with elevated levels of blood cholesterol, especially in the absence of any additional risk factors.

Just providing people with nutritional information (for example, telling them that fat and cholesterol are "bad") is no guarantee that they will change their attitudes or life-styles. Rigid diets are rarely sustained for a long time, whether the benefits are immediate (such as weight loss) or long-term (better cardiovascular health). A rational and flexible dietary alternative that requires no great sacrifice and does not create guilt for occasional or short-term indiscretions has a better chance of being accepted and followed. *Choosing Foods for a Healthy Heart* presents this alternative.

6

Dietary Cholesterol:
The Overblamed Nutrient

❦

Practically every cell in the human body—and in *all* animals, including livestock, birds, and marine animals—needs cholesterol to survive. However, like certain nutrients such as vitamins A or D, excessive long-term intake of cholesterol in some individuals may be harmful.

Dietary cholesterol does not raise the levels of blood cholesterol in everyone. As mentioned, only about 20 to 30 percent of the population seem to be cholesterol "responders," those in whom excessive dietary cholesterol raises blood cholesterol levels. For the other 70 to 80 percent, moderate-to-high dietary intake of cholesterol plays only a negligible role in raising blood cholesterol levels or in affecting cardiovascular health.

Obviously the 150–175 million Americans whose total blood cholesterol levels are desirable (below 200 mg/dl) are not all vegetarians or on cholesterol-restricted diets. Nearly all of them eat an average diet containing at least moderate amounts of cholesterol and various other fats. The reason some cholesterol "nonresponders" have elevated blood cholesterol is that other dietary and genetic factors account for their high cholesterol levels. For them, dietary cholesterol is not the culprit.

28

Cholesterol "Responders" and "Nonresponders"

Numerous studies in which volunteers have been fed several eggs daily for months or even years have failed to show a significant change in blood cholesterol levels in cholesterol "non-responders."*

Judging by all the interest in dietary cholesterol, one would think that we are eating tons of it every day. But in fact, the average intake of dietary cholesterol for Americans is 233 milligrams per day for children one to five years old, 272 milligrams per day for women, and 435 milligrams per day for men. These are hardly excessive numbers, especially for children and women. If a low intake of dietary cholesterol is so desirable, then why do 70 percent of women over the age of 45 have elevated levels of blood cholesterol even though their average daily intake is only 272 milligrams, some 10 percent below the recommendation of the American Heart Association? And why do 80 percent of women with coronary heart disease have low levels of the "good" HDL cholesterol?

Many studies in which dietary cholesterol is reduced to less than 300 milligrams per day have not shown a substantial drop in the blood level of the "bad" LDL cholesterol. In fact, studies have shown that for every 100-milligram reduction in dietary cholesterol intake, there is an average decrease of only 2.3 to 4 mg/dl in blood cholesterol! This is simply too trivial and unimpressive to justify all the fuss and publicity surrounding dietary cholesterol. Furthermore, dietary cholesterol doesn't change directly into blood cholesterol and is less important than saturated fat in raising levels of blood cholesterol.

There are several ways the body handles dietary cholesterol:

1. Normally, people absorb about 30 to 50 percent of their dietary cholesterol. When they eat foods containing a large

---

*Recently, an 88-year-old man was found to have perfectly normal blood cholesterol, even though for 15 to 20 years he had been eating about 25 eggs every day, amounting to approximately 6,000 milligrams of dietary cholesterol daily.

amount of cholesterol, most people tend to absorb a smaller portion of this dietary cholesterol from the intestine. (For example, when an elderly man who ate 25 eggs per day was studied, he could absorb only 18 percent of his dietary cholesterol.)

2. Through a "feedback" mechanism in response to dietary cholesterol and saturated fat intake, the liver automatically reduces or stops its internal production of cholesterol.

3. Under normal conditions, about 70 percent of the "bad" LDL cholesterol in the blood enters the liver through special receptors, or gates, on the surface of liver cells. Once inside liver cells, this cholesterol is converted to bile, which is discharged into the small intestine and used in the digestion and absorption of fats and fat-soluble vitamins. But in some persons whose blood cholesterol is raised in response to diet, the ability of the receptors to take LDL cholesterol out of blood circulation is genetically limited. On the other hand, in people with normal genes for LDL receptors, the number (and ability) of the liver's receptors for LDL cholesterol are significantly higher. This enables the liver to take in and convert the cholesterol into bile more efficiently. These individuals can handle LDL cholesterol normally.

4. In most people, LDL receptors are special "gates," or receiving docks, reserved for entry of the "bad" LDL cholesterol into the liver for disposal. In some people, these receptors may be defective or not fully functional, or they may tend to be more receptive to other lipoproteins than LDL. All of these receptor abnormalities can cause levels of blood cholesterol to go up. Depending on certain genetic abnormalities (or mutations) in the LDL-receptor gene, there may be as many as 180 different types of LDL receptors, each with different functional limitations. One particular genetic abnormality makes these LDL receptors less interested in LDL particles but more attracted to imposters. For example, in some cholesterol "responders," when dietary cholesterol is absorbed from the intestine, blood also picks up a special protein called apoprotein E4. This combination of cholesterol and apo E4 (see Figure 6.1) creates imposters that fool LDL receptors into allowing them to enter, as if they were the real, "bad" LDL.

FIGURE **6.1**

Structure of the LDL Imposter

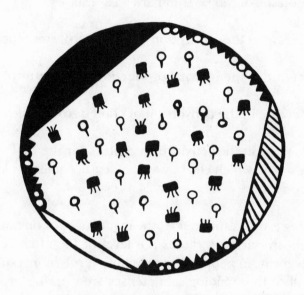

◗	**Apoprotein B**
⏺	**Apoprotein C**
◠	**Apoprotein E**
○	**Cholesterol**
▲	**Complex fats**
♀	**Cholesterol bound to a fatty acid**
⚵	**Triglycerides**

Once inside, these imposters occupy spaces reserved for circulating LDL. Because the liver cannot accommodate so many LDL particles, they have no place to go and are forced to remain in blood circulation, thus raising the blood cholesterol.

Defensive Actions

Various defensive actions that the body can take in response to dietary cholesterol can be summarized as follows:

- a decrease in the absorption of cholesterol from the intestine
- a decrease in the internal production of cholesterol by the liver
- an increase in the conversion of cholesterol to bile in the liver
- an increase in the activity of receptors for the LDL cholesterol, which clear away the "bad" cholesterol from the circulation

In cholesterol "responders," the inadequacy of one or more of these defensive actions causes the level of blood cholesterol to rise. Conversely, in people who are cholesterol "nonresponders," most or all of these biological defenses are working properly, so diet does not result in a sustained elevation of their blood cholesterol levels. These biological defenses also explain why lipoprotein levels can fluctuate in virtually everyone by as much as 20 to 25 percent from week to week.

It is incorrect to assume that blood cholesterol levels remain stable until we eat an egg. A review of 27 recent studies shows that at current levels of average dietary cholesterol intake (272 milligrams per day for women and 435 milligrams per day for men), additional intake of cholesterol causes little if any measurable change in blood cholesterol levels. Therefore, it is a mistake to be preoccupied with dietary cholesterol alone and to assume that it must be avoided at all costs.

At the present time, there is no way to determine who is a cholesterol "responder" or "nonresponder" without performing exhaustive studies usually undertaken for research purposes. However, for most of the population, an average daily cholesterol intake of 300 to 400 milligrams—equivalent to the cholesterol content of two medium-size eggs—is not associated with any undesirable side effects, especially if consumption of saturated fatty acids is reduced (see chapter 7). This is an important consideration, particularly when dealing with children or the elderly, for whom eggs and various meats provide excellent sources of nutrition.

7

Dietary Saturated Fatty Acids

Saturated fatty acids (SFA) are among the worst nutritional offenders for cardiovascular health. The potential of saturated fats to raise blood cholesterol levels is three to four times greater than that of dietary cholesterol. In addition, the specific type of fat eaten is far more important than how much.

As with cholesterol, saturated fats have "high responders"— those who will respond to dietary saturated fats with a rise in their blood cholesterol levels. On the other hand, millions of "low responders" show no appreciable change in blood cholesterol levels when they eat saturated fats. The genetic reasons for this are unclear at this time.

Saturated Fats Increase the Risk of Coronary Heart Disease

Dietary saturated fatty acids contribute to coronary heart disease in two ways:

As explained in chapter 6, most of the "bad" LDL cholesterol is eventually removed from the blood by the liver and is used to produce bile. These "bad" LDL particles enter the liver cells through specially designated receptors. In "high responders," sat-

urated fats stimulate the internal production of cholesterol, especially by the liver. In response to this high rate of cholesterol
production, liver cells cut back their LDL-receptor capacity and
many LDL particles cannot be cleared from the blood. Having no
place to go, they accumulate in the circulation and raise the level
of blood cholesterol. In effect, the body has only one way to deal
with excessive amounts of dietary saturated fats: We are dependent on our LDL receptors to do the job.

In the long run, elevated "bad" LDL cholesterol can result in
fatty streaks in the walls of the arteries, some of which can eventually change into the plaques seen in coronary artery disease. It
is doubtful that the "bad" LDL as is can actually cause any serious
harm unless it is oxidized and thus converted to a "mean" LDL.
Once saturated fats are absorbed from the intestine, they are
partly mixed in with particles of "bad" LDL. The concern is that
these newly formed LDL particles may be of the more aggressive
variety (LDL-3). Unfortunately, these LDL particles are easily oxidized, producing a "mean" LDL, which is gobbled up by white
blood cells (monocytes) in the arterial wall, where they start the
process of atherosclerosis. This potential of SFA may be even
more important than whether they raise blood cholesterol levels.

Saturated fats also increase the tendency of blood platelets to
clump and form tiny blood clots within the arteries. Although
most of these small clots will be dissolved, some gradually become
larger, eventually clogging the affected arteries (thrombosis). This
clot-producing potential of SFA is another important reason why
saturated fats are unfriendly and undesirable, whether an individual is a high or low "responder."

All Saturated Fats Are Not Equal

Some researchers believe that certain saturated fatty acids are
potentially more damaging to the arteries than others. Our foods,
however, contain a mixture of various fatty acids (see Figure 7.1),
and it is impossible to separate the neutral effects of some SFA
from the unfavorable effects of others. For example, beef fat con-

FIGURE 7.1

Various Types of Fatty Acids

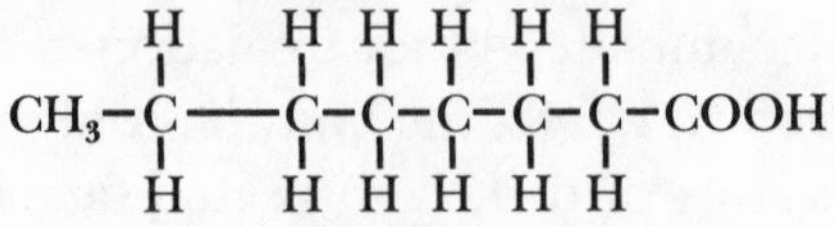

$$\begin{array}{cccccc} H & H & H & H & H \\ | & | & | & | & | \\ CH_3-C&\!\!\!-\!\!\!-\!\!\!-\!\!\!C\!-\!C\!-\!C\!-\!C\!-\!C-COOH \\ | & | & | & | & | \\ H & H & H & H & H \end{array}$$

Saturated Fat

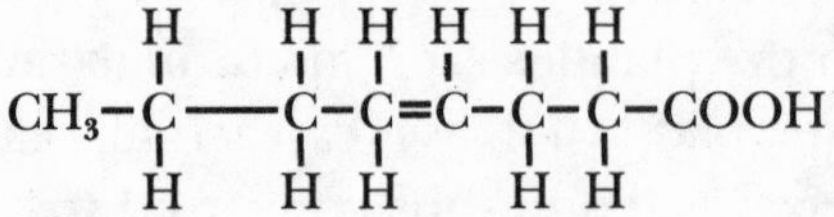

$$\begin{array}{cccccc} H & H & H & H & H \\ | & | & | & | & | \\ CH_3-C&\!\!\!-\!\!\!-\!\!\!-\!\!\!C\!-\!C\!=\!C\!-\!C\!-\!C-COOH \\ | & | & & | & | \\ H & H & & H & H \end{array}$$

Monounsaturated Fat

$$\begin{array}{ccccccc} H & H & H & H & H & H & H \\ | & | & | & | & | & | & | \\ CH_3-C&\!\!\!-\!\!\!-\!\!\!-\!\!\!C\!=\!C\!-\!C\!=\!C\!-\!C\!=\!C-COOH \\ | & & & & & & \\ H & & & & & & \end{array}$$

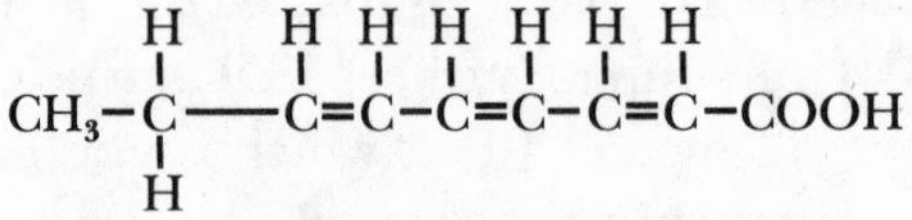

Polyunsaturated Fat

- When all the carbon molecules are fully occupied (they have *single bonds*, or −), the fatty acid is saturated.
- When the carbon molecules are not fully occupied (they have *double bonds*, or =), the fatty acid is unsaturated.
- If one carbon molecule is unsaturated, the fatty acid is *mono*unsaturated. If more carbon molecules are unsaturated, the fatty acid is *poly*unsaturated.

tains substantial amounts of an SFA called stearic acid, which does not raise the blood cholesterol. For this reason, it is called a neutral or even a "good" saturated fat. But even if stearic acid does not increase the LDL cholesterol, other saturated fats accompanying stearic acid may be unfriendly enough to increase the aggressive LDL-3 and promote its conversion to "mean" oxidized

LDL. They can also promote clot formation and thus increase the risk of coronary thrombosis and heart attack. Moreover, beef fat always contains these other undesirable saturated fats, so regular consumption of fatty red meats (but not lean red meats) is still not "heart-friendly."

Although SFA are undesirable, in the real world we cannot avoid them. Otherwise, eating becomes a nuisance and a chore instead of a pleasure. Using the CEF Index eliminates all the worries about knowing the cholesterol or saturated fatty acid content of foods.

8

Dietary Polyunsaturated
Fatty Acids

🍂

Overzealous and often misleading promotion of polyunsaturated fats occurs regularly in print, radio, and television. Popular magazines offer advice and recipes using margarines or other forms of polyunsaturated fats to promote cardiovascular health. Are these health claims fact or fiction?

Polyunsaturated Fats

There are two distinctly different groups of polyunsaturated fatty acids (PUFA), as shown in Figure 8.1:

- The omega-6 PUFA are present mostly in vegetable oils, shortenings, and margarines, and in very small amounts in some animal fats.
- The omega-3 PUFA are present in all seafood (including shellfish), some nuts (almonds, pecans, pistachios, walnuts), and in soybean and canola oils. The differences between these two groups are so vast that in some respects they are at two opposite poles.

FIGURE 8.1

Polyunsaturated Fatty Acids

$$CH_3-\underset{\underset{H}{|}}{\overset{\overset{H}{|}}{C}}-\underset{\underset{H}{|}}{\overset{\overset{H}{|}}{C}}-\overset{\overset{H}{|}}{C}=\overset{\overset{H}{|}}{C}-\underset{\underset{H}{|}}{\overset{\overset{H}{|}}{C}}-\underset{\underset{H}{|}}{\overset{\overset{H}{|}}{C}}-\underset{\underset{H}{|}}{\overset{\overset{H}{|}}{C}}-COOH$$

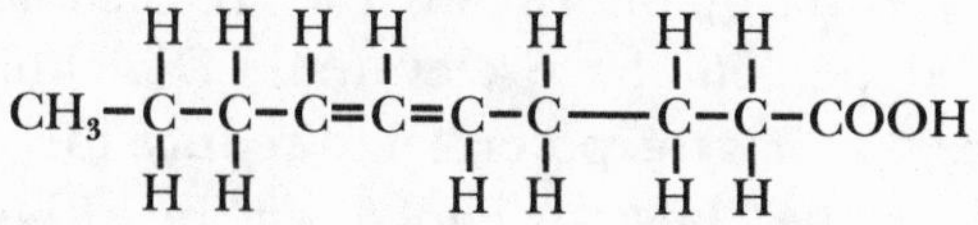

Omega 3 (n-3) Polyunsaturated Fat

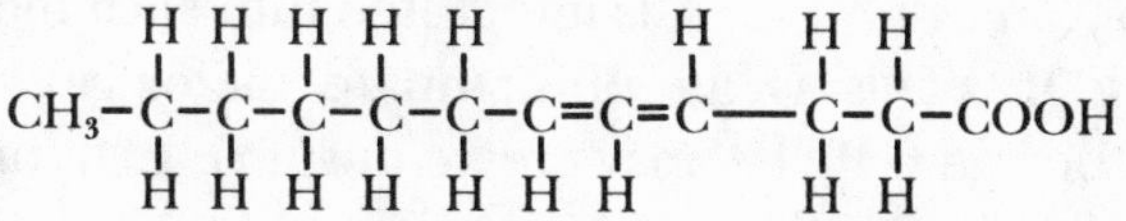

$$CH_3-\underset{\underset{H}{|}}{\overset{\overset{H}{|}}{C}}-\underset{\underset{H}{|}}{\overset{\overset{H}{|}}{C}}-\underset{\underset{H}{|}}{\overset{\overset{H}{|}}{C}}-\underset{\underset{H}{|}}{\overset{\overset{H}{|}}{C}}-\underset{\underset{H}{|}}{\overset{\overset{H}{|}}{C}}-\overset{\overset{H}{|}}{C}=\overset{\overset{H}{|}}{C}=\overset{\overset{H}{|}}{C}-\underset{\underset{H}{|}}{\overset{\overset{H}{|}}{C}}-\underset{\underset{H}{|}}{\overset{\overset{H}{|}}{C}}-COOH$$

Omega 6 (n-6) Polyunsaturated Fat

The carbon position of the first double bond (=) from the left end of the polyunsaturated fatty acid determines the omega (n-) status.

Dietary Omega-6 Polyunsaturated Fatty Acids

The role of dietary omega-6 PUFA (from vegetable oil, margarine, and vegetable shortening) in coronary heart disease is almost entirely limited to the minor effect they have in reducing the level of "bad" LDL cholesterol. Even this effect is mostly accomplished by replacing saturated fatty acids in the diet. Otherwise, excessive consumption of omega-6 PUFA has a host of undesirable side effects.

• *They reduce the level of beneficial HDL cholesterol.* Numerous studies have shown that even moderate consumption of polyunsaturated fats (less than 10 percent of total calories daily, as recommended by present dietary guidelines) has the adverse potential to reduce the blood level of "good" HDL cholesterol (especially its cardioprotective subclass, HDL-2).

As mentioned earlier, in people with coronary heart disease, low levels of the "good" HDL cholesterol are far more common than elevated "bad" LDL cholesterol. Nearly 80 percent of individuals with CHD have abnormally low HDL cholesterol, while about 20 to 30 percent have elevated LDL cholesterol. Any dietary practice that has the potential to reduce the "good" HDL cholesterol cannot be "heart-friendly" or "heart-healthy," especially for those who already have low levels of HDL cholesterol.

• *They may convert the "bad" LDL to the "mean" LDL.* A portion of dietary omega-6 PUFA is integrated into each molecule of the "bad" LDL. This is an unfortunate biological combination, because omega-6 PUFA may create unstable LDL molecules that can more easily oxidize and be converted to "mean" cholesterol. Although at present we do not know how frequently or in which individuals this process occurs, this harmful effect alone may well outweigh any beneficial effects omega-6 PUFA have in lowering the "bad" LDL cholesterol.

• *Hydrogenation produces undesirable trans fatty acids.* The hydrogenation of commercial vegetable oils converts liquid oils to solids; it also protects these oils from getting rancid (oxidized) and at the same time adds texture and flavor. During hydrogenation, especially in the processing of stick margarines and vegetable shortenings, as much as 30 percent of the PUFA is converted to undesirable trans fatty acids (see Figure 8.2).

Trans fatty acids (TFAs) are even worse than SFA because they not only raise blood levels of the "bad" LDL cholesterol but also lower the "good" HDL cholesterol level. More important, they help to convert the LDL cholesterol into the highly atherogenic oxidized LDL. In a recent study 239 persons admitted to Boston area hospitals with their first heart attack were compared to 282 "controls." Those with the highest intake of TFA had nearly a 2½ times greater risk of having a heart attack. Another recent study estimated that regular consumption of an average amount of trans fatty acids (such as the use of margarines, shortenings, and a "Western" diet) can increase the risk of having a heart attack by about 27 percent.

• In the United States, the negative cardiovascular impact of

FIGURE 8.2

Geometric Frame of Fatty Acids

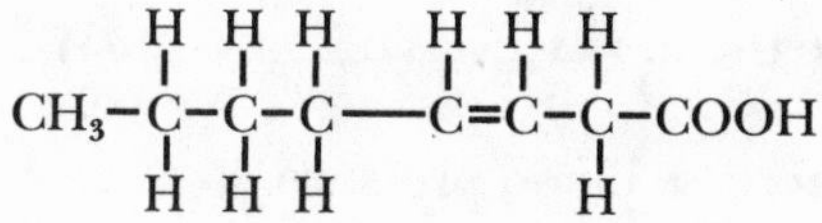

A Cis Fatty Acid

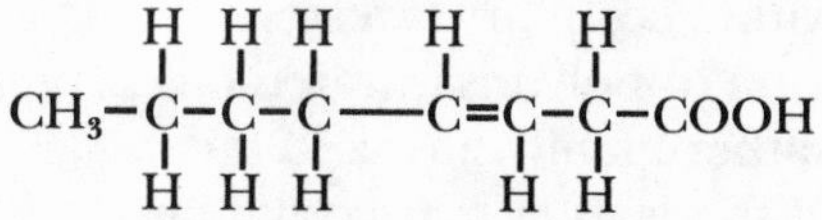

A Trans Fatty Acid

The positions of the hydrogen atoms on the unsaturated carbons (double bonds) determine the cis or trans status. If the hydrogen atoms are on one side of the unsaturated carbon, it is a cis; if they are on both sides, it is a trans fatty acid.

trans fatty acids in processed vegetable fats is not considered when P/S (PUFA/SFA) ratios are calculated. Because of this important omission, such ratios provide limited nutritional information. Since the Food and Drug Administration (FDA) does not require the labeling of foods for their trans fatty acid content, or for the presence of other hydrogenation by-products, it is likely that such information will continue to be omitted from product labels.

• *Processing can produce harmful saturated fats.* Another area of concern with hydrogenation of vegetable oils is the production of small amounts of three saturated fatty acids (arachidic, behemic, and lignoceric). Even in small quantities, these saturated fats can be harmful to the inner wall of the arteries.

• *They may interfere with the body's immune system.* Diets enriched with omega-6 polyunsaturates, especially linoleic acid (the main

---

Undesirable Side Effects of Omega-6 Polyunsaturates

- They reduce the blood levels of "good" HDL cholesterol.
- They may increase blood pressure.
- Within the LDL particles they are readily oxidized to form a "mean" cholesterol.
- They promote clumping of blood platelets and clot formation within coronary arteries.
- Hydrogenation of polyunsaturated oils produces small amounts of atherogenic saturated fats.
- In processed foods, they may contain up to 30 percent trans fatty acids, which are far worse than saturated fats.
- They may cause the formation of gallstones.
- They suppress the function of T lymphocytes and therefore decrease immunity.
- In animals, they may promote colon and breast cancer.
- They may counteract some benefits of omega-3 PUFA.

PUFA in soybeans and in corn, sunflower, and safflower oils), may suppress various functions of T lymphocytes, the white blood cells that fight infection. This is an important consideration, since many diseases can develop when immunity is reduced.

- *They may promote certain cancers.* A number of experimental studies in various animals fed a diet enriched with omega-6 PUFA show increased rates of breast and colon cancer. Of course, every time an animal study provides certain information, we cannot jump to the conclusion that the findings are relevant to humans. However, since older people are likely to have a reduced immune response as well as a higher risk of developing various cancers, they should seriously consider reducing the consumption of polyunsaturated vegetable oils. Moreover, since children and young adults have many years of exposure to high doses of these polyunsaturates, they too should be cautious in their consumption of omega-6 polyunsaturated fats.

• *They can increase the risk of heart attack.* An enormously important side effect of omega-6 PUFA, and especially trans fatty acids, is their potential to increase the risk of heart attack and stroke. This side effect is brought on by the conversion of omega-6 PUFA within the body, especially platelets, into chemical compounds (such as arachidonic acid) that cause constriction of the arteries, clumping of blood platelets, and clot formation within coronary or brain arteries.

• *Omega-6 PUFA inhibit omega-3 PUFA.* Omega-6 PUFA in vegetable oils can counteract certain beneficial effects of omega-3 polyunsaturates in seafood. You defeat the purpose of eating seafood if you fry it in (or cook it with) so-called heart-healthy and no-cholesterol vegetable fats, including margarines.

What Should the Consumer Do?

As noted above, chemical changes in hydrogenated vegetable oils, margarines, and shortenings may have a number of negative health effects (see box). Clearly they are not "hearty" or "heart-

---

**Products That Contain Omega-6
Polyunsaturated Fatty Acids**

- Deep frying oils*
- Vegetable spreads*
- Margarines*
- Vegetable shortenings*
- Corn oil
- Sunflower oil
- Safflower oil
- Peanut oil
- Processed Peanut butter*
- Soybeans

*May contain up to 30 percent harmful trans fatty acids

healthy" substitutes for other fats (as they are often advertised). In fact, current recommendations that dietary PUFA can be increased to about 10 percent of daily energy intake are too liberal. At present, the average daily intake of omega-6 PUFA in the United States is about 5 to 6 percent of dietary energy. This is a reasonable level of consumption and is the equivalent of about 15 grams (½ ounce) of vegetable shortening or margarine per day.

Linoleic acid (the major omega-6 PUFA) is an essential fatty acid the human body needs but cannot make. However, we need less than 2 grams of linoleic acid a day. There is no need to consume large amounts of any fat, whether it comes from a cow or from plants such as corn or peanuts, especially if they are processed (hydrogenated).

Dietary Omega-3 Polyunsaturates from Seafood

Dietary omega-3 polyunsaturates are present primarily in all seafood (see Table 8.1), as well as in some plant sources such as almonds, pistachios, pecans, walnuts, and soybean and canola oils. The role of omega-3 polyunsaturates, or any other nutrient, should not be viewed only from the standpoint of blood cholesterol levels; this limited view ignores other biological effects of nutrients on the cardiovascular system and the whole body. The vast multipurpose benefits of omega-3 polyunsaturates in seafood are so impressive that regular consumption of seafood is one of the most important preventive measures against cardiovascular events.

• *Omega-3 PUFA reduce the risk of developing atherosclerosis.* Omega-3 polyunsaturates can help prevent the development of atherosclerosis and coronary heart disease in three ways:

a. *They improve blood lipids.* Eating seafood will not cause a dramatic change in the "good" HDL or the "bad" LDL cho-

TABLE 8.1

Fatty Acid Composition of Seafood

	Total Fat	SFA	MUFA	Omega-3 PUFA	Cholesterol
Fish					
Mackerel, Atlantic	13.9	3.6	5.4	2.6	80
Trout, lake	9.7	1.7	3.6	2.0	48
Trout, rainbow	3.4	0.6	1.0	0.6	54
Herring, Atlantic	9.0	2.0	3.7	1.7	60
Tuna, bluefin	6.6	1.7	2.2	1.6	38
Salmon, Atlantic	5.4	0.8	1.8	1.4	74
Salmon, coho	6.0	1.1	2.1	1.0	60
Bluefish	6.5	1.4	2.9	1.2	59
Bass, striped	2.3	0.5	0.7	0.8	80
Bass, freshwater	2.0	0.4	0.7	0.8	59
Pompano	9.5	3.5	2.6	0.6	50
Shark	1.9	0.3	0.4	0.5	44
Halibut	2.3	0.3	0.8	0.5	32
Perch	2.5	0.6	0.9	0.4	80
Cod	0.7	0.1	0.1	0.3	43
Flounder	1.2	0.3	0.2	0.4	46
Shellfish					
Mussels	3.6	0.9	0.9	1.0	36
Clams	2.2	0.6	0.4	0.9	36
Oysters, eastern	2.6	0.7	0.5	0.9	47
Squid	1.8	0.8	0.1	0.8	280
Crab	1.3	0.2	0.2	0.6	71
Shrimp	1.2	0.3	0.3	0.5	157

SFA = saturated fatty acids
MUFA = monounsaturated fatty acids
PUFA = polyunsaturated fatty acids

lesterol. However, in the majority of individuals with elevated "bad" VLDL (very-low-density lipoproteins) and triglycerides, omega-3 PUFA from seafood can improve these abnormalities, at times dramatically. As triglycerides are lowered, the HDL levels may rise in many of these individuals.

b. *They reduce the production of the "mean" LDL.* There is a large body of evidence suggesting that the "bad" LDL must undergo some modification of its structure and function before it can become the "mean" LDL. Omega-3 polyunsaturates from seafood may reduce or block the oxidation of LDL and its conversion to a "mean" cholesterol.

Omega-3 polyunsaturates in seafood are also the only nutrients that may reduce the blood level of the other "mean" lipoprotein, Lp(a). For many individuals, especially African-Americans, Lp(a) may contribute more to plaque deposits than the "bad" LDL or VLDL cholesterols do.

c. *They reduce the inflammation and thickening of arteries.* Omega-3 fatty acids help the body produce numerous anti-inflammatory substances. These enormously helpful substances reduce the risk of injury to, or inflammation of, the arterial wall caused by various coronary risk factors. The less injury there is to the arterial wall, the less inflammation, scarring, thickening, and eventual narrowing of the arteries. Nearly all of these benefits are independent of blood cholesterol levels and would be ignored if we focus on changes in blood cholesterol only.

• *Omega-3 PUFA reduce the risk of clot formation within arteries (or heart attack).* Unlike the polyunsaturates in vegetable oil, omega-3 PUFA from seafood not only prevent the development of hardening of the arteries but may also help to prevent clot formation (thrombosis) within coronary and cerebral arteries. This effectively reduces the risk of heart attacks and certain types of stroke. A recent study examined the effects of various dietary interventions in over 2,000 persons who suffered a previous heart attack. They were assigned to one of three dietary regimens: (1) a low-cholesterol, low-fat diet; (2) a high-fiber diet; and (3) a diet that increased fatty fish intake (two or three meals per week containing fish such as mackerel, kippers, salmon, sardines, or trout). After only two years, the group that ate fish regularly had nearly one-third less overall mortality than did the other two groups. This significant benefit was independent of any change in blood cholesterol levels, since there was only a 3.6 percent drop in blood cholesterol for the group during this period. What is more important is that the amount of fish in the diet was relatively small, about 10 ounces per week.

• *Omega-3 polyunsaturates reduce the risk of reclogging the arteries after coronary bypass surgery or angioplasty.* As noted, for clogging of the arteries to occur and take hold, there must be some initial damage or injury to the inner wall of these arteries. Unfortunately, during coronary bypass surgery, especially during balloon dilatation of atherosclerotic arteries (balloon angioplasty), there is almost always new, and at times, substantial damage to the thin inner lining of the arteries (endothelium). This often creates cracks and sores, and the new injured areas are susceptible to clot formation. In up to 45 percent of people treated with angioplasty, the procedure-related injury will result in partial or complete reclogging and narrowing of the arteries.

There is evidence that eating seafood or certain types of fish oil helps to prevent reclogging of the arteries after coronary angioplasty. In a recent study, the best results were achieved when increased consumption of omega-3 PUFA was started several weeks *before* angioplasty and continued indefinitely. Six months after the procedure, when coronary arteries were radiographed and compared to those of patients who were not treated with omega-3 PUFA, the risk of reclogging was reduced by as much as one-third to two-thirds. More important, eating just more than 8 ounces (227 grams) of seafood per week was comparable to taking a large number of certain fish-oil capsules every day. On the other hand, dietary intake of other fats, including cholesterol, saturated fat, omega-6 PUFA, or total fat, had no effect on the rate of reclogging.

The beneficial effects of omega-3 polyunsaturates do not

become apparent until they reach certain concentrations in various body cells, including cells in the arterial wall, and platelets. This usually requires eating seafoods regularly—three or four times a week for several weeks. For this reason, eating a piece of fish or a tuna sandwich once every week or two is not likely to provide a significant benefit. Moreover, a large number of people with CHD who require angioplasty or coronary artery bypass surgery have high blood levels of the "mean" lipoprotein (a). As noted, elevated Lp(a) levels are not responsive to conventional dietary recommendations but may be lowered by increasing the intake of omega-3 PUFA. Obviously, if you need emergency angioplasty or bypass surgery, "pretreatment" with omega-3 polyunsaturated fats is not an option. However, if it is an elective procedure, starting omega-3 PUFA four to six weeks beforehand may help prevent reclogging of the arteries. The important point is that only relatively small amounts of seafood omega-3 PUFA are required for many of these highly desirable cardiovascular benefits.

Frequent consumption of omega-3 polyunsaturates from seafood can reduce the risk of intravascular clotting (coronary or cerebral thrombosis) in several ways. For example, omega-3 PUFA become a component of newly formed blood platelets, partially replacing omega-6 in these cells. This substitution transforms the function and the personality of platelets: Instead of producing chemical substances that constrict the arteries and clump the platelets to form intravascular clots, the beneficial new platelets containing omega-3 PUFA produce substances that dilate the arteries and prevent clotting. Moreover, the blood levels of various clotting factors (especially fibrinogen) are also decreased, further lowering the risk of intravascular clotting.

• *Omega-3 polyunsaturates may reduce irregularities of heart rhythm.* Several studies have suggested that the presence of high levels of omega-3 PUFA within the heart muscle may significantly reduce the risk of severe life-threatening heart rate irregularities. However, additional studies are required to confirm these preliminary reports and to see whether consumption of seafoods can reduce the need for "anti-arrhythmia" drugs.

• *Omega-3 polyunsaturates reduce blood pressure.* Recent studies have shown that long-term consumption of seafood raises the blood levels of omega-3 PUFA, which can result in a significant reduction of blood pressure. For hypertensive individuals, this is clearly a bonus (see box page 50).

Omega-3 Polyunsaturates from Plant Sources

Although omega-3 polyunsaturated fats from plant sources are far more desirable than other vegetable oils, they do not have the same important benefits as the omega-3 PUFA in seafood. The reason for this is that omega-3 PUFA from plant sources are almost exclusively linolenic acid, which has a slightly different chemical makeup from the omega-3 polyunsaturates in seafood. Within the human body, the omega-3 PUFA from plant sources are partially converted to the seafood variety. However, this is usually a very slow process.

Vegetables, fruits, and certain kinds of nuts are excellent sources of high-quality nutrients, including vitamins and minerals. The presence of monounsaturates (avocado, olives, nuts) and omega-3 polyunsaturates (green vegetables, herbs, and some types of nuts such as almonds, pistachios, pecans, and walnuts but not peanuts or cashews) makes them particularly desirable for cardiovascular as well as overall health.

Fish-oil Extracts: Risks and Benefits

Some fish-oil extracts can lower blood triglycerides and the "bad" VLDL cholesterol levels by as much as 40 to 45 percent. The maximum benefit requires 8 to 9 grams (about 20 capsules!) of omega-

**Cardiovascular Benefits of
Omega-3 Polyunsaturates in Seafood**

1. They reduce the risk of developing atherosclerosis by:
    - Reducing inflammation and narrowing of the arteries
    - Reducing "bad" VDL and triglycerides
    - Reducing "mean" lipoproteins
    - Reducing blood pressure
2. They reduce the risk of intravascular clotting (thrombosis), which can result in heart attacks and strokes, by:
    - Reducing the aggregation of blood platelets and their release of chemicals, which may cause clotting and constriction of the arteries
    - Altering the function of blood platelets so that they release chemicals that dilate the arteries
    - Reducing the blood levels of various clotting factors
    - Making red blood cells more pliable so they can squeeze through narrowed or very small arteries to deliver oxygen
    - Reducing the risk of irregular heart rhythm and sudden death
    - Reducing the risk of reclogging of the arteries after coronary bypass surgery or angioplasty
    - Reducing the extent of heart muscle damage that occurs after heart attacks (by reducing toxic free radicals—see chapter 13, "Iron")

**Sources of Omega-3
Polyunsaturated Fatty Acids**

- Seafood, including shellfish
- Green leafy vegetables—herbs (very small amounts)
- Some nuts—almonds, pistachios, pecans, and walnuts
- Soybeans and soybean oil
- Canola oil

3 polyunsaturates per day. However, smaller doses (2 to 3 grams per day) may have some slight benefit. In some studies, salmon and tuna oils have also been shown to lower the "bad" LDL cholesterol. On the other hand, pollock oil and some commercially available fish-oil extracts do not lower LDL and may even raise the level of harmful apoprotein B. Another concern is that many commercially available fish oils can aggravate diabetes and worsen blood cholesterol abnormalities in diabetic individuals.

Many popular fish-oil extracts contain more than 30 percent saturated fatty acids, which are extremely atherogenic. Different fish-oil extracts also have variable concentrations of trans fatty acids. From the cardiovascular standpoint, these saturated fats and trans fatty acids are the worst offenders.

All fish oils are not the same, however. The composition of their beneficial fatty acids (omega-3 polyunsaturates), as well as their concentration of trans and saturated fatty acids, plays a significant role in how a fish-oil extract behaves. Furthermore, certain fish oils, including cod-liver oil, contain highly unstable polyunsaturated fats that are readily oxidized in the body into very undesirable chemicals. Still, the addition of supplemental vitamin E can reduce this potential.

These important differences in safety and efficacy illustrate the fact that many fish-oil extracts are not safe, and some may even be hazardous. The differences in composition may also explain why salmon and tuna oils are far more beneficial to cardiovascular health than many other commercially available fish oils.

In comparison to fish-oil extracts, seafood contains extremely low amounts of saturated fats (less than 1 percent). Seafood is also practically free of trans fatty acids and other undesirable fatty acids. These distinct advantages make a strong case for eating seafood rather than taking fish-oil extracts. However, as noted earlier, persons undergoing coronary artery bypass or angioplasty can reasonably consider using fish oils (salmon or tuna) accompanied by supplemental vitamin E. In this situation, the overall benefits of these fish oils may outweigh their side effects in aggravating diabetes in those who already suffer from that disease.

Side Effects of Omega-3 Polyunsaturates in Seafood

Unlike omega-6 polyunsaturates, which are available in large quantities in commercially available vegetable oils, vegetable shortenings, and various margarines, the omega-3 PUFA are present in very small quantities in seafoods, some nuts, and vegetables. It is important to remember that naturally occurring omega-3 obtained from seafood is different from processed, commercially available fish oils. From a practical standpoint, the possibility of any side effects from the consumption of omega-3 polyunsaturates in seafood is nonexistent.

Theoretically, because omega-3 PUFA reduce the potential for clotting of the blood, the risk of bleeding may be increased in some people who take fish-oil supplements. However, this has never been known to happen, even during various surgical procedures. Fish-oil extracts are distinctly different from seafood, and they do have some side effects, as described earlier. These side effects are caused by the presence of impurities and various amounts of saturated or trans fatty acids that accumulate during the processing of fish-oil extracts.

Omega-3 polyunsaturated fats from seafood may provide a broad range of health benefits and protection against coronary heart disease. Eating three to four seafood meals per week (including shellfish) is one of the most effective means of reducing the risk of heart attack. Some fish-oil supplements such as salmon or tuna oils may have a beneficial role in protecting against clogging of coronary arteries after bypass surgery. However, they should not be substituted for seafood.

9

Dietary Monounsaturated
Fatty Acids

❦

A large body of evidence suggests that long-term consumption of monounsaturated fatty acids (MUFA) as a partial replacement for saturated fats may lower the "bad" LDL cholesterol level and the risk of coronary heart disease. Studies have also shown that monounsaturates may help reduce blood pressure, one of the major risk factors for heart attack and stroke.

Recent studies have shown that diets high in olive oil (72 percent MUFA) result in a significant decrease in the blood level of the "bad" LDL cholesterol. This is apparently accomplished by stimulating and increasing the activity of LDL receptors in the liver. The abundance of these receptors seems to accelerate the removal of LDL particles from the blood, lowering their blood levels.

Olive oil is unique among vegetable oils because it also contains a beneficial substance called squalene. Squalene, independent of olive oil's monounsaturated fatty acid, may have a role in preventing the formation of oxidized LDL ("mean" cholesterol).

The relatively low concentration of saturated fats in both olive oil (14 percent) and canola oil (6 percent) is another benefit. For most stick margarines and vegetable shortenings, the saturated fat content is much higher—23 to 30 percent. Just as important is the absence of trans fatty acids in olive and canola oils.

Injury to the inner wall of the arteries (the endothelium) may be a prerequisite for coronary heart disease. Saturated fats have the tendency to perpetuate this injury. Monounsaturates, as substitutes for dietary SFA, may reduce this additional risk, especially over a long period of time.

Diets rich in monounsaturated fatty acids can make LDL cholesterol more stable and therefore less likely to be oxidized into a "mean" cholesterol. This is an enormously important benefit of MUFA, and along with other advantages, it may explain the substantially lower rates of coronary heart disease in certain populations. People in the Mediterranean region, for example, use far more olive oil than any other fat.

Benefits of
Monounsaturated Fatty Acids (MUFA)

- They are safe substitutes for both saturated fats and omega-6 polyunsaturates in the diet.
- They lower blood pressure (and therefore reduce the risk of heart attack and stroke).
- They reduce the risk of clot formation (thrombosis) within coronary arteries.
- They lower the level of the "bad" LDL cholesterol in the blood while increasing the level of the "good" HDL cholesterol.
- Unlike omega-6 PUFA, they reduce the conversion of the "bad" LDL to the oxidized "mean" LDL.
- Unlike processed vegetable oils, they do not contain toxic by-products of hydrogenation such as trans fatty acids.
- Long-term use of monounsaturates such as olive or canola oils may reduce the risk of coronary artery disease.

Reduced Risk of Clot Formation

There is also a strong possibility that MUFA reduce the risk of clot formation (thrombosis) within coronary arteries, thereby decreasing the risk of heart atacks.

Recent studies show that the diets of three groups—strict vegetarians, ovolactovegetarians (those who eat eggs and dairy products), and persons who eat fish but no red meat—often contain more total fat (mostly MUFA and PUFA) than the average American diet. Yet in all three groups, the levels of blood cholesterol, the risk of coronary heart disease and various cancers are far more favorable than for those who eat the usual Western diet.

Because of the vast beneficial effects of monounsaturated fats (see box) and their versatility for use in preparing all kinds of foods, dietary MUFA are the most suitable, all-purpose oils for all people. From a practical viewpoint, they are the ideal substitutes for saturated fats and omega-6 polyunsaturates.

10

Dietary Fiber

❧

Dietary fiber refers to the nonstarchy complex carbohydrates in plant foods. Although fiber is considered nonnutritive because it is not digested or absorbed in the small intestine, it is in fact broken down in the large intestine and partially absorbed. Not all dietary fiber is the same; some is *soluble* and some is *insoluble* in the intestinal juices. Vegetables and fruits contain large amounts of both kinds of fiber. Soluble fiber is present in legumes, oats, and nuts. Wheat bran is the most widely recognized source of insoluble fiber.

Does Dietary Fiber
Lower Blood Cholesterol Levels?

Many studies reporting the cholesterol-lowering effect of fiber have involved large supplemental doses of soluble fiber consumed three or four times per day, an impractical amount for most people. In many of these studies, subjects were also placed on low-cholesterol, low-fat diets, so it is difficult to attribute any benefit to fiber alone.

One recent study examined the response of normal volunteers (without elevated blood cholesterol levels) to high and low amounts of supplemental fiber. Oat bran by itself showed little or no cholesterol-lowering effect beyond that accomplished by reducing saturated fat in the diet. A detailed study of strict vegetarians and ovolactovegetarians also showed that when allowance was made for reduced intake of saturated fats and increased consumption of monounsaturates and polyunsaturates, the very-high-fiber intake of vegetarian diets had no effect on blood cholesterol levels.

An analysis of 10 recent studies detailing the cholesterol-lowering effects of oat bran showed that long-term use of these products may at best reduce blood cholesterol levels by an average of only 5 to 10 mg/dl.

How Dietary Fiber Works

The role of dietary fiber in lowering blood cholesterol is mostly the result of reducing and replacing saturated fatty acids in the diet. However, dietary fiber may have a small independent role in lowering the "bad" LDL cholesterol. To some extent, soluble fiber (or possibly one of its active ingredients, beta-glucan) absorbs the bile in the small intestine and eliminates it with the waste. To replace the lost bile, the liver converts some of the circulating "bad" LDL cholesterol into new bile. This increased conversion of LDL to bile may result in a small drop in the blood cholesterol level. But even if dietary fiber could reduce blood cholesterol through other mechanisms, the overall reduction would still be trivial.

On the basis of available data, it appears that the role of dietary fiber in reducing the risk of coronary heart disease is relatively minor and indirect (i.e., through a small reduction in LDL cholesterol). However, dietary fiber lacks any favorable effect on the level of "good" HDL cholesterol and can have many uncomfortable digestive side effects—gas, bloating, diarrhea, and cramps, especially when consumed in excessive amounts. Long-term use of soluble fiber at high doses can also reduce the absorption of iron and cause iron-deficiency anemia. It can also interfere with the absorption and effectiveness of certain medications.

In the real world, it is not always easy to know the composition of dietary fibers (soluble or insoluble). For example, some psyllium products contain as much as 70 percent soluble fiber, whereas oat bran has only 16 percent. Many vegetables, fruits, and

TABLE 10.1

Total Dietary Fiber of Fruits and Vegetables
(grams per 3.5-ounce portion unless otherwise indicated)

Fruits	Fiber	Vegetables	Fiber
Figs, dry (5)	12	Baked beans	9
Prunes, dry (5)	8	Kidney beans	7
Apricots, dry	8	Navy beans	6
Blackberries	7	Lima beans	5
Raspberries	5	Peas	4
Apricots, fresh (5)	4	Corn	4
Dates (5)	4	Sweet potato	3
Banana (1)	4	Carrot, large (1)	3
Pear (1)	4	Potato, large, with skin (1)	3
Mango (1)	3	Broccoli (1 stalk)	3
Apple (1)	3	Tomato, large (1)	3
Nectarine (1)	3	Brussels sprouts	2
Orange, large (1)	3	String beans	2
Raisins (¼ cup)	3	Bean sprouts	2
Peach, large (1)	2	Asparagus	2
Plums (3)	2	Summer squash	2
Strawberries	2	Zucchini	2
Blueberries	2	Cabbage	2
Cherries	1	Kale	2
Grapes	1	Onions	2
Grapefruit (1)	1	Cauliflower	2
Cantaloupe (½ cup)	1	Celery	1
Honeydew (½ cup)	1	Mushrooms	1
Watermelon (2 cups)	1	Lettuce	1
		Spinach	1
		Radishes (5)	1
		Peppers	1
		Cucumber, large (1)	1

grains contain adequate amounts of both soluble and insoluble fiber (see Table 10.1). There is also a good deal of overlap between the effects of various sources of dietary fiber. In addition, it is always preferable to eat a variety of fruits, vegetables, and grains rather than consuming supplemental soluble fiber.

11

Dietary Salt

In some individuals, excessive salt intake may aggravate a tendency toward high blood pressure. There are, however, several qualifying points to consider. Although the diet consumed by most Americans and Europeans contains approximately 10,000 milligrams (equivalent to two teaspoons) of salt per day, not everyone who consumes this much is hypertensive. In fact, it is unlikely that salt, even at present levels of consumption, can actually cause hypertension in those not already predisposed to this condition.

"Responders" and "Nonresponders"

Among people with hypertension, only 15 to 20 percent may be salt "responders." And even in this group, salt restriction alone is often inadequate for the control of their hypertension. This is especially true among African-Americans, even though they tend to be more "salt-responsive" than whites.

In a recent comprehensive, international study of the relation between dietary salt and hypertension, it was found that dietary salt intake showed a tendency to be associated with hypertension only among older persons. In another study, among more than 30,000 U.S. male health professionals aged 40 to 75 years, dietary salt intake was not found to contribute to high blood pressure, at least during a four-year follow-up.

One potentially harmful aspect of even moderate salt restriction is that such a diet may cause a significant rise in blood pressure in approximately 15 percent of hypertensives ("reverse responders"). Moreover, salt restriction can result in weakness and fatigue, decreased sexual potency in men, and sleep disturbances. And because low-salt or salt-free diets have little personality or taste, they may contribute to malnutrition, especially in older persons.

Since an estimated 60 million Americans have high blood pressure, we can assume that about 10 to 12 million of them might benefit somewhat by reducing their salt intake. On the other hand, the rest of the population, with or without high blood pressure, would not benefit appreciably from this dietary modification. In fact, approximately 10 million hypertensives—along with countless others—might even be harmed by it.

Daily Salt Intake

It is reasonable to argue that the average daily salt intake of 10,000 milligrams is much more than the body needs (about 1,000 milligrams per day). Yet, there are an endless number of things we don't need but which we enjoy because they improve our quality of life. Moreover, long-term adherence to a low-salt diet, as with any other rigid dietary restriction, is very low. In a recent study (in New York), only one-quarter of those on low-salt diets were able to stay on them for any length of time.

One-third of our daily salt intake is provided by natural foods, one-third comes from processed foods, and one-third is added during cooking or at the table. Breads, rolls, and crackers supply most of the dietary salt, followed by processed meats such as hotdogs, luncheon meats, and ham. On the other hand, added salt in many frozen vegetables can amount to no more than 50 to 100 milligrams per serving, or about 1 percent of our total daily salt intake. As with many other nutrients, it is the long-term excesses that may have undesirable effects in some individuals. Eating one or two salted foods per day is barely of any consequence.

High blood pressure is a major risk factor for cardiovascular complications, and lowering one's blood pressure reduces the frequency of these events. But we cannot conclude that because salt may aggravate high blood pressure in some individuals, the non-hypertensive population should limit salt in their diets. As with dietary cholesterol intake, we have overemphasized the negative effects of salt.

A recent German study showed that only about 15 percent of persons with hypertension are "salt-responsive," but more important, salt restriction resulted in significant increases in the "bad" LDL cholesterol and triglyceride levels, especially among "reverse responders."

Other recent studies suggest that high blood pressure in adolescents, obese adults, diabetics, and African-Americans is more likely to be salt-responsive. However, even for them, only a modest reduction of dietary salt intake to approximately 4 to 6 grams per day (equivalent to avoiding "salty" foods and processed meats) is sensible. Increasing dietary calcium and potassium at times may improve the effectiveness of modest salt restriction (moderate amounts of potassium are found in lean red meat, poultry, seafood, green vegetables, cereals, potatoes, bananas, oranges, prunes, avocados, and the commercially available salt substitutes). However, a recent randomized study at the University of Texas at Houston showed that after three years a low-salt, high-potassium diet had no beneficial effect on controlling blood pressure.

In short, dietary salt intake has only a relatively minor role in coronary heart disease for some people with hypertension. For millions of those with normal blood pressure, restricting salt intake has no short- or long-term benefit and may turn eating into a boring and tasteless exercise.

12

Proteins, Carbohydrates, Vegetables, and Fruits

There is no evidence to suggest that carbohydrates or proteins have a significant impact on the process of atherosclerosis. It is true that substituting carbohydrates for fat (especially for saturated fatty acids) may help reduce LDL cholesterol. However, this benefit is the result of lower levels of SFA in the diet, not higher intake of carbohydrates.

Effects of Carbohydrates

Numerous studies have shown that although eating large amounts of complex carbohydrates (pasta, bread, various grains) may reduce the "bad" LDL cholesterol level, it may also lower the level of "good" HDL cholesterol in the blood, at times by as much as 30 to 40 percent. More important, the blood level of apo A-1, the cardioprotective component of HDL cholesterol, is reduced by about 20 percent. This is not a trivial matter for the 70 to 80 percent of Americans for whom the risk of CHD from low levels of HDL cholesterol is far greater than from elevated levels of LDL or total blood cholesterol.

For millions of diabetic, overweight, or obese persons, and those with elevated blood triglycerides as well, excessive intake of carbohydrates is undesirable. In fact, a high-carbohydrate diet can increase the "bad" VLDL cholesterol and triglycerides by as much as 35 percent. Very high carbohydrate intake can also contribute to the ineffectiveness of insulin in the blood, a condition known as insulin resistance. Recent data offer strong evidence that insulin resistance is a major risk factor for CHD. Under these circumstances, cutting down on carbohydrates makes sense, especially simple carbohydrates (candies, cookies, cakes) and "light," complex carbohydrates (white bread, white pasta, white rice, and potatoes), which are readily broken down into simple carbohydrates in the intestine. Moreover, many of these carbohydrates contain hidden amounts of very undesirable ingredients such as butter, cream, vegetable shortening, and coconut oil.

Another concern is that a portion of digested carbohydrates will be converted to fatty acids (and stored fat). In both humans and herbivorous animals (including cattle, poultry, etc.) a substantial part of these newly formed fatty acids is palmitic acid, which is perhaps the most atherogenic fatty acid. But perhaps even more alarming is the recent finding that consumption of large amounts of carbohydrates will actually increase the amount of LDL-3 cholesterol, which is the "bad" and "unfriendly" subclass of LDL.

Obesity and Carbohydrates

There is no doubt that obesity, especially the abdominal variety, is a major risk factor for various types of blood lipid abnormalities and coronary heart disease. Weight reduction—cutting down on caloric intake while getting regular exercise, or by correcting any existing metabolic disorder—frequently improves abnormalities in the blood lipids. However, losing weight by dieting alone does not have a significant effect on blood lipids. Moreover, even mild-to-moderate obesity is associated with enlargement and thickening of the wall of the heart, both of which can lead to heart failure and other cardiovascular complications. Very obese individuals of both sexes are 15 to 17 times more likely to have an enlarged heart than are lean persons. Weight reduction gradually reduces this enlargement and thickening of the wall of the heart.

In terms of overall health, moderate amounts of complex carbohydrates and proteins are excellent nutrients, but from the standpoint of coronary heart disease, they are neutral. Nearly all very-low-fat diets are based on the premise that 80 percent or more of dietary energy should come from carbohydrates. There is simply no justification for increasing dietary carbohydrates beyond 50 to 60 percent of daily caloric intake. Excessive dietary carbohydrates may increase blood levels of the "bad" LDL-3 and VLDL cholesterol and triglycerides, reduce the level of beneficial "good" HDL cholesterol, contribute to insulin resistance, aggravate diabetes, and cause obesity.

The Effects of Vegetables, Fruits, and Grains

With the exception of coconut and palm products, all vegetables, fruits, and grains are excellent nutrients. Many vegetables, especially greens, are extremely low in fat, but as much as 50 percent of their fatty acids are the heart-pleasing and healthful omega-3 polyunsaturates. Romaine lettuce, chicory, spinach, broccoli, cauliflower, brussels sprouts, cabbage, kale, parsley, leeks, and green beans are especially high in omega-3 polyunsaturates. Walnuts, pecans, almonds, pistachios, and soybeans also have 6 to 10 grams of omega-3 polyunsaturates in each 3.5-ounce edible portion. Although avocados are approximately 17 percent fat, they contain less than 3 percent saturated fats, over 11 percent monounsaturated fat, and negligible amounts (3 percent) of polyunsaturates. Another important factor is that vegetables, fruits, and grains, by providing a feeling of fullness, may reduce your total caloric intake and may also "displace" omega-6 polyunsaturates and saturated fats in the diet.

Vegetables and fruits are also terrific sources of many vitamins and minerals. Several population studies have shown far less cardiovascular mortality in people who eat plenty of fresh fruits and green vegetables. Although the abundance of vitamins C and especially E may be responsible for this cardioprotective effect, numerous other substances could also be involved. For example, long-term use of beta carotene (present in practically all vegetables and fruits) may significantly reduce the risk of a new heart attack or stroke in those with preexisting cardiovascular disease. However, there is no evidence that beta carotene can prevent the development of atherosclerosis or coronary heart disease in healthy people.

Vegetables, fruits, and grains provide a wide range of nutrients that may reduce the risk of coronary heart disease. A vast number of these nutrients are *not* available in multivitamin or mineral supplements, either over-the-counter or by prescription. "I'll take my vitamins instead" is no substitute for eating fruits, vegetables, and grains.

13

Vitamins and Minerals

In the United States, we spend an estimated $5 billion a year on vitamin and mineral supplements. These are mostly wasteful and unnecessary products that provide very little health benefit. In addition, there is no convincing evidence that the usual doses of multivitamins or Recommended Daily Allowance (RDA) of various vitamins or minerals has any role in prevention or treatment of coronary heart disease and atherosclerosis.

The Effects of Vitamins

When the "bad" LDL cholesterol is oxidized, it becomes especially harmful to the inner wall of coronary arteries. Several recent studies suggest that vitamins C and E may partially block the oxidizing of LDL. However, at RDA levels for the two vitamins, this "antioxidant" effect is probably too small to be useful.

Whether larger doses of vitamin E (up to 800 to 1000 milligrams, or 20 to 25 times the RDA) or vitamin C (500 to 1,000 milligrams, or about 8 to 16 times the RDA) have any cardioprotective role is not clearly established. A recent study from Britain showed that chest pain (angina) due to coronary artery disease was 2.5 times more common among persons with the lowest blood levels of vitamin E than among those with the highest levels. However, the frequency of anginal attacks was unrelated to blood levels of vitamins A or C, or to beta carotene (a close relative of vitamin A).

Some population studies suggest that high doses of vitamin C (1,000 milligrams per day) may lower the levels of the "bad" LDL cholesterol or increase the levels of the "good" HDL cholesterol. But such effects are usually limited to people who have vitamin C deficiency to begin with, a disorder that is almost nonexistent in developed countries.

To determine the relevance of "antioxidant" vitamins (A, C, and E) to coronary heart disease, 16 European populations with different mortality rates from CHD were recently studied. Annual CHD death rates per 100,000 population ranged from 66 in the Catalonia region of Spain to 470 in the Karelia region of Finland. This study found that cross-cultural differences in CHD mortality were primarily attributable to variations in vitamin E levels in the blood. The association with vitamin E levels was even stronger than differences in blood cholesterol, blood pressure, or other vitamins combined.

Two recent U.S. studies presented in fall 1992 at the annual meeting of the American Heart Association, which involved more than 130,000 U.S. male and female health professionals with no history of cardiovascular problems, showed that vitamin E lowered the risk of CHD in women by 40 percent and in men by 26 percent. In both studies, participants took a daily supplement of more than 100 mg of vitamin E for two or more years.

It is assumed that supplemental vitamin E, even in those who are not vitamin-E deficient, prevents the oxidation of LDL particles by free radicals (see the section on the role of iron and oxygen-free radicals in this chapter). In effect, vitamin E assumes or supplements the antioxidant function of "good" HDL.

At present, on the basis of all available evidence, for persons with high blood LDL or low HDL levels, especially in those with coronary artery bypass surgery, supplemental vitamin E at daily doses of up to 800–1,000 mg may be worth considering. At these doses there are no harmful side effects, and theoretically there is the potential for cardioprotective benefit.

Recent studies suggest that vitamin C can improve the effectiveness of vitamin E by converting oxidized vitamin E back to its natural (and active) form. Eating modest portions of fruits and vegetables should provide an adequate amount of vitamin C for this purpose, as well as plenty of beta carotene and vitamin A so that supplemental doses are not necessary.

Niacin

Large doses of niacin, such as 3,000 to 6,000 mg per day (or greater than 100–200 times the RDA), have been used to lower blood levels of the "bad" LDL cholesterol and increase the "good" HDL cholesterol. At these doses, niacin ceases to be a vitamin and in effect becomes a drug, with side effects severe enough that over 50 percent of patients stop taking it. (These side effects can include flushing, diarrhea, nausea, lack of energy, and, on rare occasions, liver damage.)

Nondietary niacin, starting with small doses and gradually increasing the dose over many weeks, lowers the "bad" LDL cholesterol, but more important, it raises the levels of the "good' HDL by over 30 percent. This increase is almost entirely accounted for by the more than 100 percent increase in cardioprotective HDL-2, which moves a greater amount of cholesterol from the blood to the liver and therefore reduces the risk of coronary heart disease. Niacin may also be effective in reducing the blood level of the "mean" lipoprotein (a), which is highly unresponsive to other available drugs.

Because niacin (especially some time-release or sustained-release forms) may have toxic side effects, large doses should not be taken without a physician's strict supervision. However, if niacin is used properly—and as a drug—it has many beneficial and cardioprotective effects. Taking niacin with meals (and along with one aspirin, if aspirin is not otherwise contraindicated) should reduce some of the side effects, especially facial flushing.

Other Vitamins

Recent studies suggest that as many as 20 to 40 percent of individuals under age 60 with hardening of the arteries have an inherited disorder in which blood levels of a group of proteins collectively referred to as homocyst(e)ine are elevated. Although it is not clear as to how homocyst(e)ine causes atherosclerosis and coronary heart disease, there is some evidence that it may damage the inner wall of the arteries. Three vitamins in the B group—vitamin B_6, folic acid, and vitamin B_{12}—are necessary co-factors in the breakdown of homocyst(e)ine. Moderate to high doses (10 to 50 times the RDAs) of these three vitamins expedite and increase the breakdown of this complex protein and therefore lower the blood levels (if they are abnormally high). There is at present no long-term experience using these vitamins to prevent or treat atherosclerosis, with or without elevated homocyst(e)ine levels.

Minerals

There is no direct relationship between minerals and coronary artery disease or atherosclerosis. However, minerals play an important role in the function of the heart muscle as well as the tone of blood vessels. In this regard, abnormal levels of potassium, magnesium, and calcium can cause serious irregularities in heart rhythm, especially in people with preexisting heart problems.

Recent studies have shown that a modest increase in potassium intake significantly reduces the risk of stroke and heart attack in some hypertensive persons. (Potassium is present in moderate quantities in fruits, vegetables—especially leafy greens and potatoes—all meats including seafood, all legumes, and salt substitutes.) The beneficial response to potassium is more pronounced among hypertensive individuals who have a high renin blood level. Renin, which is produced by the kidneys, can be readily measured by a blood test.

Although some earlier studies had suggested that supplemental magnesium and calcium may lower blood pressure, recent studies have not confirmed these findings. Both minerals have important roles in regulating the heart's rhythm, but they are not involved directly in promoting or preventing CHD. However, once plaques are formed in the arterial wall, invariably some calcium will also be deposited within these plaques, contributing to arteriosclerosis (hardening of the arteries). In fact, calcification of the arteries is the indisputable evidence of arteriosclerosis.

Iron

The evidence is mounting that iron may play an important role in the development of coronary artery disease. A recent study suggests that the lower levels of iron in premenopausal women may be just as important as higher estrogen levels in explaining the difference in CHD death rates for men and women. Women lose a good deal of iron each month through menstruation, so they have much lower levels of stored iron in their bodies than do men. This may explain in part why the risk of CHD in women before menopause is about one-third that of men the same age. However, after menopause, when women stop losing iron through monthly periods and their bodies accumulate more iron, the gap for mortality from CHD between men and women closes rather rapidly.

Free Radicals

Although the accumulation of iron in many organs (heart, lungs, brain, pancreas) can cause serious damage, its role in coronary artery disease is indirect, as a catalyst or facilitator. At any given time, countless biological activities are taking place in every cell in our bodies. During many of these activities, small amounts of very unstable substances called free radicals are produced. Free radicals can potentially damage everything they come into contact with, including the very cells in which they are produced.

Fortunately, we have "balancing" antidotes in our cells, and most of these free radicals will be neutralized as soon as they are produced. Some free radicals have unstable oxygen atoms (oxygen-free radicals). Molecules of iron can convert oxygen-free radicals into more toxic and unstable compounds that readily convert the "bad" LDL into the "mean" oxidized LDL and can also directly damage the heart muscle.

Some pioneering studies now suggest that, in fact, we should not be too eager to correct all iron "deficiencies," since we might be trading in a minor condition for a significantly increased risk of coronary heart disease. On the other hand, severe iron deficiency does have a number of undesirable consequences, such as a lowered immune system and decreased resistance to infections, lowered exercise and work performance, and abnormal behavioral and neuropsychological patterns.

Clearly, the practice of taking iron pills for fatigue, stress, and low energy (most of which have nothing to do with "iron-poor blood") may indeed be unsafe and even harmful. A recent study from Finland (where the prevalence of CHD is among the highest in the world) suggested that for each milligram of daily iron intake there was a 5 percent increase in the risk of heart attack. The risk was highest among those with elevated LDL cholesterol, affirming the role of iron as an oxidant of LDL cholesterol. On the other hand, two recent U.S. studies (the National Health and Nutrition Examination Survey and the U.S. Physicians Study) did not show any significant association between blood-iron levels and CHD.

The accumulating body of evidence strongly suggests that injudicious use of iron supplements without a physician's supervision or documented need must be discouraged. This is especially applicable to those who have other risk factors for CHD, especially abnormal blood cholesterol levels.

14

Tea, Coffee, and Alcohol

Tea, coffee, and alcohol are not nutrients, but they are consumed by a vast number of people on a regular (and frequent) basis. Very often their cardiovascular benefits or harmful effects are misunderstood, exaggerated, or subject to biased reporting.

Tea

There is no evidence to suggest that tea has any effect, one way or the other, on the process of atherosclerosis and CHD. Because of its small amount of caffeine (approximately 20 to 25 milligrams per cup, as compared to 100 to 120 milligrams per cup of coffee), it may have some stimulatory effect on the heart muscle. However, this is a negligible effect and has no connection with coronary arteries or cardiovascular diseases.

Coffee

The health risks of coffee and caffeinated beverages have been debated for years. Numerous studies dealing with and clarifying the cardiovascular effects of coffee have been reported. In a study from Finland, people who drank eight cups of *boiled* coffee daily for four weeks demonstrated a significant rise in their blood cholesterol levels, whereas drip-filtered coffee had no effect on cholesterol. More recently, investigators from the Netherlands isolated an oily substance in boiled coffee that contributes to elevated cholesterol levels. This substance, which can seep through during boiling, is unrelated to caffeine or other ingredients in coffee.

In a recent U.S. study of more than 45,000 men 40 to 75 years old, moderate coffee consumption was not associated with any increased risk of cardiovascular events. Although only about 3 percent of the subjects in the study drank six or more cups of coffee per day, even in that subgroup the relative risk of cardiovascular diseases did not increase. However, several other recent studies suggest that drinking more than five to six cups of coffee (regular or decaffeinated) may indeed increase the risk of heart attack, especially for men under 60.

The oily extract of coffee beans that can seep through during boiling is thought to contain a cholesterol-raising substance. This extract is invariably removed with paper filters; furthermore, it has no relevance if one is drinking moderate amounts of coffee (fewer than five cups per day). It is not known whether this oily substance seeps through metal or plastic filters, or if it is present in espresso coffee. However, since the volume of espresso consumed in this country is very small, it is unlikely that it has any cholesterol-altering effect for most Americans.

Excessive coffee drinking may occasionally cause minor irregularities in the heart rate. However, moderate amounts of coffee have no appreciable effect on heart rhythm in normal persons or in those with preexisting coronary heart disease. (This excludes the harmful role of smoking, which is a common practice among many coffee drinkers.) Similarly, although heavy coffee drinking may increase one's blood pressure slightly, several recent studies have reported lower blood pressures in regular coffee drinkers who consume low or moderate amounts of the beverage.

Alcohol

Reports from Australia, Britain, France, and the United States have shown that regular consumption of small to moderate amounts of alcohol (two to three cocktails, two to three glasses of wine, or two to three beers per day) may decrease the risk of coronary heart disease by as much as 45 percent. Alcohol provides this cardioprotective benefit in several ways. Small-to-moderate amounts of alcohol may slightly raise the blood level of the "good" HDL cholesterol. Alcohol may also reduce the risk of clot formation (thrombosis) within the coronary arteries by altering the functions of blood platelets and the amount of various clotting factors present in the blood. A British study suggested that because alcohol improves the response of muscles and other organs to insulin, the body requires much less insulin to metabolize carbohydrates. It is known that excessive amounts of insulin in the blood can damage the inner lining of coronary arteries. For this reason, lower levels of circulating insulin (brought about by alcohol, weight loss, or exercise) will produce a response that is always favorable to the cardiovascular system.

Wine and Coronary Heart Disease

Recent data from the World Health Organization show that the French have a much lower death rate due to coronary heart disease than other Western industrial countries. For example, the annual CHD death rate per 100,000 men in Toulouse, France, is 78, compared to 182 in Stanford, California, and 380 in Glasgow, Scotland. Although the rates in women are substantially lower than in men, they still follow a similar trend; the numbers are 11, 48, and 132, respectively.

There are, of course, a number of explanations for this remarkable French advantage. The diet in Toulouse is Mediterranean, with lots of bread, vegetables, and fruits and very little butter but quite a bit of cheese and wine. However, various statistical analyses suggest that the wine may also have a significant cardioprotective role. Of course, higher levels of physical activity and their lack of genetic predisposition are also additional reasons for a lower rate of CHD in this population.

It is highly unlikely that wine (red or white), consumed more heavily by French than by Americans or the British, has a unique virtue other than its alcoholic content. On the other hand, there is a possibility that some ingredients in red wine (other than alcohol) may also have cardioprotective benefits. Since grape skins are used extensively in making red wine, some chemicals such as polyphenols and phytoalexins, which are plentiful in grape skin, will seep through and remain active in the wine. Polyphenols are potent antioxidants that may play a role in preventing oxidation of LDL and damage to coronary arteries. Phytoalexins can raise HDL cholesterol and reduce the tendency of platelets to aggregate and form intravascular clots.

It has been shown that for several hours after eating, especially after fatty meals, circulating blood becomes more "hypercoagulable" (more likely to form intravascular clots). Alcohol, by acting on blood platelets, decreases the clotting ability. Because wine is mostly consumed during meals, it may provide a beneficial anticlotting effect during the more vulnerable few hours after eating.

Alcohol also improves the response of muscle cells to insulin, so that carbohydrates can be more efficiently metabolized. Insulin allows muscle cells to break carbohydrates down into carbon dioxide and water and store what is not used within the muscle cells as glycogen. Alcohol improves the storage phase of insulin action, thereby reducing the need for overproduction of insulin by the pancreas. Evidence has shown that excessive amounts of insulin can directly (as well as indirectly) damage the inner wall of coronary arteries.

Drinking wine with meals (as French do) is therefore more likely to provide cardioprotection than drinking beer or cocktails during "happy hours" (as Americans and many other Westerners do).

Light Versus Heavy Drinking

A recent French study showed that light-to-moderate alcohol consumption increased the level of beneficial apoprotein A-1, responsible for the "heart-friendly" action of the "good" HDL cholesterol. However, as drinking increased, apo A-1 decreased progressively, even though the level of the "good" HDL continued to rise. This is an enormously important finding; we cannot assume that since small amounts of alcohol raise the "good" HDL cholesterol level, larger amounts are even more beneficial for cardiovascular health. In fact, by reducing the level of apoprotein A-1, excessive drinking may increase the risk of coronary heart disease and heart attack—regardless of its effect on HDL-cholesterol levels. Moderate-to-heavy drinking also increases the levels of triglycerides and the "bad" VLDL cholesterol, both of which are major risk factors for CHD.

Although light drinkers may have a lower incidence of coronary heart disease or high blood pressure, more than two to three drinks per day may contribute to hypertension. Aside from high blood pressure, the risk of stroke increases dramatically in heavy drinkers. Among people who suffer a stroke, heavy drinking is twice as common in men and seven times as common in women than it is in the general population.

Regular and excessive drinking of alcohol damages the heart muscle in nearly one-half of heavy drinkers. Alcohol is a major cause of heart-rate irregularities and sudden death in persons under 65 years of age. One study of sudden unexpected deaths in women without known heart disease showed that 40 percent were related to alcohol abuse. Several reports have shown similar data for men. Most of these sudden deaths have been due to acute irregularities in the heart rate.

Clearly, no one should recommend regular and heavy use of alcohol for the purpose of raising the "good" HDL cholesterol or reducing the rate of heart attacks. However, for most adults (excluding pregnant women), there is no evidence that one or two drinks per day is harmful to the heart. And when alcoholic beverages are taken with meals, they may even provide some cardiovascular benefit. Beyond this narrow range, William Shakespeare was right: "First the man takes a drink, then the drink takes a drink, the drink takes the man."

15

Pitfalls of Current
Dietary Recommendations

❧

Many of the present dietary recommendations of the American
Heart Association and the National Cholesterol Education Program are rational, sensible, and useful (see Table 15.1). However,
there are a number of major misconceptions that make long-term
adherence to such recommendations difficult, unpleasant, and
unnecessary.

Misconceptions

Present dietary recommendations are based on the assumption
that low-fat, low-cholesterol diets lower blood cholesterol levels
and therefore reduce the risk of cardiovascular diseases. However, no food's health effects can be judged solely on the basis of
its cholesterol or fat content, or what it may or may not do to the
blood levels of the "bad" LDL cholesterol. Such a narrow focus
ignores the exceedingly diverse or even competing roles of different nutrients.

Between 70 and 80 percent of people with coronary heart disease have low levels of the "good" HDL cholesterol, and only 20
to 30 percent have elevated levels of the "bad" LDL cholesterol.
Even in the latter group, an elevated level of "bad" LDL is fre-

TABLE 15.1

Current Dietary Recommendations for High Blood Cholesterol*

Recommended daily intake of selected nutrients
as a percentage of total calories

Nutrient	Step 1 Diet	Step 2 Diet	Step 3 Diet
Total fat	<30	<25	<20
Saturates	<10	<7	<5
Polyunsaturates	Up to 10	Up to 10	Up to 10
Monounsaturates	10–15	10–15	10–15
Carbohydrates	50–60	50–60	60–70
Protein	10–20	10–20	10–20
Cholesterol	<300 mg/day	<200 mg/day	<100 mg/day
Calories	To achieve and maintain a desirable weight.		

< = less than
*Recommendations of the National Cholesterol Education Program and the American Heart Association

quently not the only risk factor. These people may also have high levels of the "mean" lipoprotein (a), or low levels of the "good" HDL cholesterol. Furthermore, as noted earlier, only 1 to 1.5 percent of those with elevated blood cholesterol have coronary heart disease. The remaining 99 percent either do not have CHD, or if they do, it does not cause any problems. Low-fat, low-cholesterol diets have very little relevance to these individuals.

The average daily cholesterol intake in the United States is currently 272 milligrams for women and 435 milligrams for men, levels that do not justify a preoccupation with dietary cholesterol alone. Reducing average cholesterol intake by 100 to 200 milligrams per day will lower blood cholesterol levels by only about 4 to 8 mg/dl, which in a person with a high blood cholesterol level is practically negligible.

To see how a one-dimensional focus on total blood cholesterol or LDL cholesterol can be misleading, the case of one 31-year-old

TABLE 15.2

Abnormal Lipoproteins with "Desirable" LDL

Abnormal Lipoproteins with "Desirable" LDL	*Subject (mg/dl)*	*"Desirable" range (mg/dl)*
Triglycerides	210	<120
Total cholesterol	185	<200
LDL cholesterol	116	<130
VLDL cholesterol	42	<30
HDL cholesterol	27	<45
Cholesterol/HDL ratio	6.85	<4 to 1

computer engineer is a good example. Several members of this man's family, including his father and a brother, died prematurely of coronary heart disease. Although the man's total blood cholesterol and the "bad" LDL cholesterol levels were both "normal," his triglycerides and VLDL cholesterol levels were high; his level of "good" HDL cholesterol was very low and provided no protection against atherogenic lipids, including the VLDL and the aggressive LDL-3 particles. All this information combined shows that he would be at considerable risk for premature cardiovascular events, even though his LDL cholesterol was "normal."

Why Present Dietary Recommendations Are Inadequate

Five recent U.S. and three British studies have shown that long-term adherence to present dietary recommendations is unlikely to provide significant protection against cardiovascular events:

1. In the Toledo, Ohio, Exercise and Diet Study in 1990, subjects were placed on a restricted low-fat, low-cholesterol diet for six months. At the end of the study, there was only a 4 percent reduction in the level of the "bad" LDL cholesterol but a dis-

heartening 12 percent reduction in the "good" HDL cholesterol. Because each 1-mg/dl decrease in HDL can increase the risk of coronary heart disease by about 4 percent, any disproportionate lowering of the HDL cholesterol is counterproductive and dangerous.

2. In the Chicago Women's Study, a group of women went on a strict low-fat, low-cholesterol diet for five months (Step 3 of the NCEP-AHA). At the end of the study period, the "bad" LDL cholesterol was lowered by 11 percent, but triglycerides went up by about 30 percent. More important, levels of cardioprotective HDL-2 progressively decreased during the course of the diet, and by the fifth month they were 35 percent below what they were before the strict low-fat, low-cholesterol diet was started.

3. In a Stanford, California, study, the subjects followed the American Heart Association Step 1 Diet for one year. Both men and women showed no improvement in the levels of the "bad" LDL, the "good" HDL, or apoprotein A-1, the cardioprotective protein of HDL.

4. In a Seattle, Washington, study, individuals with coronary heart disease and elevated blood cholesterol levels were randomly placed on two treatment programs. One group followed a low-cholesterol, low-fat diet while the second group followed a similar diet but also received appropriate cholesterol-altering drugs. After two and a half years on this diet alone, there was only a trivial (7 percent) reduction in levels of LDL cholesterol. However, there was no improvement in the levels of the "good" HDL cholesterol or apoprotein A-1. More important, in many their coronary artery disease actually progressed, causing heart attacks in some. By contrast, those who followed a similar diet and took cholesterol-altering drugs showed a far greater improvement in their blood lipids—and they had a 73 percent reduction in the rate of cardiovascular events.

5. In a New York study, the effectiveness of one of the modern cholesterol-altering drugs was compared in two groups of individuals who had elevated blood cholesterol levels. One group was placed on a rigid low-fat, low-cholesterol diet (the Step 2 diet of the American Heart Association); the other group was placed on a high-fat, high-cholesterol diet. Both groups were then given an identical dose of a cholesterol-lowering drug daily for several weeks. In *both* groups, LDL cholesterol levels dropped by 30 percent, while the beneficial HDL cholesterol increased by about 8 percent.

Obviously, no one is suggesting that we should be on a high-fat, high-cholesterol diet, or that we should use cholesterol-altering drugs indiscriminately. In fact, there is no argument that we should all reduce our intake of saturated fat and trans fatty acids and use cholesterol-altering drugs very selectively. Nevertheless, these and many other studies show that in many people a reduction of dietary fat and cholesterol is totally inadequate to treat or prevent CHD. For a vast number of people, this limited approach grossly underestimates the importance of a host of other nutritional and life-style factors.

Limited Benefits of Lifetime Dietary Restrictions

Millions of adults have "borderline high" cholesterol levels (200 to 240 mg/dl) without any symptoms or other associated risk factors. Since there is no study to show the benefits of lifelong, rigid, low-fat, low-cholesterol diets for such low-risk individuals, computer models have been used to predict any possible benefits.

Three separate computer models have shown that when we account for the impact of other risk factors, these lifetime dietary restrictions offer practically no benefit. For example, restricted diets may delay the onset of coronary heart disease by only a few months (in those who would have developed it anyway) or increase life expectancy by a few days to a few months. Are these modest returns worth a lifetime of frustration, dietary hardship, and deprivation?

There are also millions of people who are borderline overweight. Do we have a social or biological mandate to urge everyone to trim down to an arbitrary weight limit? Even if we succeed in these intrusive measures, we would convert a vast number of healthy people into lifelong "patients."

A great deal of evidence suggests that for slight to moderate elevation of LDL cholesterol without other major risk factors, strict dietary interventions or the use of cholesterol-altering drugs in both men and women are in fact inappropriate.

Very-Low-Fat and No-Cholesterol Diets

If current dietary recommendations (like Steps 2 and 3 of the NCEP) were not impractical and rigid enough, recently a more restrictive and almost impossible very-low-fat, cholesterol-free diet has received a lot of publicity. This is a complete vegetarian diet, with no animal products except egg whites and one cup of nonfat milk per day. Dietary fat is reduced to less than 10 percent of calories per day, and it is cholesterol-free. No caffeine is allowed. The recommendation of the diet is based on the results of a one-year study involving 22 overweight patients with severe coronary artery disease. They were strictly supervised and made other life-style changes as well.

After one year on this program, they showed a significant reduction in their "bad" LDL cholesterol levels, but there was no improvement at all in the levels of "good" HDL cholesterol or apoprotein A-1. On average, there was also a very small (2.2 percent) improvement in the narrowing of their coronary arteries. On the other hand, nearly 40 percent of the control group (those who were not on the program) also showed less clogging in the coronary arteries. Patients who strictly followed the experimental regimen had fewer episodes of chest pain (angina). However, improvements in patients' symptoms were unrelated to this minimal reduction in the narrowing of the coronary arteries. In fact, it is doubtful that small improvements (2 to 3 percent) in the diameter of coronary arteries would have a meaningful benefit. What *is* responsible for improved cardiovascular health is a package of life-style changes—giving up cigarettes, stress management, exercise, weight loss, control of blood pressure, improving various lipid abnormalities, and altering other risk factors.

Numerous studies have shown that very-low-fat diets are more consistent in lowering the beneficial HDL cholesterol than the harmful LDL. An erroneous argument by the proponents of the very-low-fat, low-cholesterol diets is that lowering the level of the "good" HDL cholesterol in the blood is not so bad as long as it is offset by a lower level of the "bad" LDL cholesterol. Unfortunately, what is decreased by these diets is the cardioprotective component of the HDL cholesterol, at times by over 60 percent. Still, we do not yet know which component of the "bad" LDL is lowered—the small particles (LDL-3), which are the real culprits, or the larger-size particles (LDL-1), which may be harmless. One function of the HDL is to remove and transport cholesterol from arteries and other tissues to the liver. Another function of HDL is to prevent or reduce the oxidation of the "bad" LDL (which becomes the "mean" oxidized LDL). At low levels, the HDL may fail to accomplish these tasks. This is a serious problem, especially in those who have already accumulated cholesterol and fat in their arterial walls and in those with low HDL levels.

Another major flaw of the very-low-fat, low-cholesterol diets is that it is not total dietary fat but rather the *type* of fat that is relevant to cardiovascular health or disease. As explained earlier, recent studies have shown that monounsaturated fats (olive and canola oils) not only reduce the LDL cholesterol level but also increase the level of cardioprotective HDL cholesterol. Perhaps even more important, they substantially reduce the conversion of the "bad" LDL to the "mean" cholesterol. Rigid very-low-fat diets also deprive people of the vast benefits and cardioprotective actions of omega-3 polyunsaturated fats in seafood (see chapter 8).

Studies of vegetarians who consume very high amounts of dietary fat, mostly monounsaturates and polyunsaturates, have shown remarkably desirable lipoprotein-cholesterol patterns, as well as very low rates of CHD. Similar observations have also been confirmed in numerous studies of nonvegetarians and those Mediterranean populations with a high intake of dietary fat. Although Greeks and many other Mediterranean groups obtain 40 percent (or more) of their dietary energy from fat, they have one of the lowest rates of coronary heart disease. According to present dietary recommendations, however, they have been doing it wrong all these centuries! In Greek and other Mediterranean diets, monounsaturated fat in the form of olive oil is the primary source of dietary fat intake, not the high levels of omega-6 PUFA and saturated fat that are common in Western diets. In the United States, Mormons who abstain from smoking and alcohol and who exercise regularly are half as likely to die from cardiovascular events and cancers as average Americans are. Yet their total fat intake is not significantly different from that of the general population.

The Need for a New Approach

Many decades ago we used extremely rigid dietary approaches in diabetics because we had not discovered insulin or other effective oral drugs to control their disease. We forbade even a pinch of salt and drastically limited fluid intake for patients with various heart conditions because we had no cardiac medications. We placed patients with tuberculosis in sanatoriums, hoping the "air" would cure them, at a time when we had no antituberculosis drugs. All of these practices are now obsolete and have no place in nutritional and medical management of such disorders. Rigid, very-low-fat, cholesterol-free diets should not be promoted for the 100 million Americans with elevated blood cholesterol or the 6 million with coronary heart disease. Such methods ignore quality-of-life issues and make people slaves to their diets and to inflexible and often very costly programs—all for minimal health benefits. The ends here do not justify the means.

Prevention and treatment of hardening of the arteries and coronary heart disease should be directed toward all risk factors, including various abnormalities of the blood lipids. Reducing fat and cholesterol in the diet without considering the important beneficial roles of other dietary factors such as monounsaturates, omega-3 polyunsaturates from seafood, various vitamins and minerals, etc., is inappropriate. People eat foods, not individual nutrients. Numerous studies also show that long-term compliance with rigid diets is rare, even in persons who receive intensive initial instructions and show a favorable early response. *Choosing Foods for a Healthy Heart,* on the other hand, presents a new and practical approach to cardiovascular health for all ages, including children and older people.

16

The CEF Index: A Novel Approach to Nutrition

Many nutrients in our daily diet have profound effects on cardio-vascular health and disease. The majority of these biological and cardiovascular effects are often independent of whether they alter the blood cholesterol level. Foods have multiple ingredients with a variety of functions. Today's understanding of how different nutrients work requires consideration of all their biological functions for an effective and rational approach to cardiovascular health.

The CEF Index

The CEF Index provides a comprehensive and accurate tool for estimating the total cardiovascular effect of any given food. In this new system, the impact of all major nutrients, not merely choles-terol or saturated fats, is given proportional representation. The nutrients measured in the CEF Index are cholesterol, saturated fats, monounsaturated fats, different types of polyunsaturated fats (including omega-3 and omega-6 PUFA), salt, dietary fiber, carbohydrates, proteins, vitamins, and minerals. This broad system of computing and defining the cardiovascular effects of foods, or the CEF Index, required four years of research and the review of more than 1,500 scientific works relating to cardiovascular risk factors, nutrition sciences, and food technology.

How the CEF Index Works

The most important and unique feature of the CEF Index is that at a glance you can gain a broad and meaningful understanding of the cardiovascular effects of foods (CEF). Each nutrient is assigned a score from −3 to +3 on the basis of its overall cardiovascular impact. If a nutrient lowers the risk of cardiovascular disease, it is assigned a proportional minus (−); if the nutrient increases the risk of cardiovascular disease, it receives a plus (+) score. So the CEF Index of any given food is the sum of all its major nutrients, whether these ingredients are cardioprotective (minus), neutral (zero), or undesirable (plus).

In this system for basic cardiovascular protection, the total *daily* CEF Index of all foods and snacks should remain below +30. In fact, the lower the CEF Index, the better. For example, a 3.5-ounce (100-gram) serving of barbecued ribs has a CEF Index of +31, whereas a 3.5-ounce portion of baked, grilled, or broiled trout has a CEF Index of −1.

To provide an idea of how the CEF Index is calculated for each food, the CEF formula is presented in Table 16.1. This table is for information only, since the computed and ready-to-use CEF indexes of nearly one thousand items are listed in Tables 16.2 through 16.13.

How to Create a CEF Index for Any Food Not Listed

Every now and then you may find that a food is not listed in Tables 16.2 through 16.13. Almost always, you can find another food very close to it, or with similar main ingredients. With a little bit of creative comparison, you should be able to come up with an approximate CEF Index for that food. For example, if you are preparing lasagna with ricotta and mozzarella cheeses and ground beef, you have three main ingredients plus the pasta. To figure out an approximate CEF Index for this meal, add up the CEF indexes for all the main ingredients found in the tables, then divide the total by the number of the main ingredients (averaging). In the case of the lasagna, the approximate CEF Index for each 3.5-ounce portion is:

$$[(+14) + (+23) + (+17) + (0)] \div 4 = +13$$

$$[\text{Ricotta} + \text{Mozzarella} + \text{Ground Beef} + \text{Pasta}] \div 4 = +13$$

Eating should always be pleasurable and interesting, and not based on fixed menus or limited choices. The CEF Index allows you to choose nutritious as well as heart- and palate-pleasing meals at home or away from home. Try to make sure that your total daily CEF Index for all foods and snacks does not exceed +30.

TABLE 16.1

CEF Index for Each 3.5-Ounce (100-Gram) Portion

CEF Index = (CH + SFA + S)
+ (MUFA + Omega-6 PUFA + Omega-3 PUFA + DF)

CH = 100 milligrams of cholesterol	= +1
SFA = 1 gram of saturated fatty acids	= +2
S = 1,000 milligrams of salt	= +1
MUFA = 3 grams of monounsaturated fatty acids	= −1
Omega-6 PUFA = 5 grams of omega-6 PUFA (vegetable fats)	= −1
Omega-3 PUFA = 1 gram of omega-3 PUFA (seafood source)	= −3
Omega-3 PUFA = 2 grams of omega-3 PUFA (plant source)	= −1
DF = 10 grams of dietary fiber	= −1

Carbohydrates, proteins, and vitamins or minerals present in foods are considered neutral, or 0, in the CEF Index.

TABLE 16.2

CEF Indexes of Oils and Spreads
(per 2 tablespoons)

Coconut oil	+52	(92% SFA, 80% as C10–C16‡)
Palm kernel oil	+46	(82% SFA, 76% as C10–C16)
Butter	+34	(63% SFA, 44% as C10–C16)
Cocoa butter	+32	(61% SFA, 34% MUFA)
Vegetable shortening*	+28	(27% SFA, 35% trans fatty acids)
Palm oil	+24	(50% SFA, 46% as C10–C16)
Beef tallow	+22	(46% SFA, 47% MUFA)
Lard	+20	(42% SFA, 47% MUFA)
Duck fat	+15	(33% SFA, 50% MUFA)
Margarine, stick*	+14	(23% SFA, 15% trans fatty acids)
Chicken fat	+13	(30% SFA, 45% MUFA)
Cottonseed oil	+12	(26% SFA, 54% omega-6 PUFA)
Margarine, soft*	+7	(17% SFA, 10% trans fatty acids)
Mayonnaise*	+6	(14% SFA, 49% omega-6 PUFA)
Soybean oil	+2	(15% SFA, 54% omega-6 PUFA, 7% omega-3 PUFA)
Corn oil	+2	(13% SFA, 58% omega-6 PUFA)
Sunflower oil	+2	(12% SFA, 68% omega-6 PUFA)
Peanut oil†	+2	(14% SFA, 50% MUFA, 32% omega-6 PUFA)
Olive oil	+1	(14% SFA, 72% MUFA)
Safflower oil	0	(9% SFA, 78% omega-6 PUFA)
Canola oil	−6	(6% SFA, 10% omega-3 PUFA, 62% MUFA)

SFA = saturated fatty acids
MUFA = monounsaturated fatty acids
PUFA = polyunsaturated fatty acids
*Contains trans fatty acids, which are more harmful than SFAs (see chapter 8).
†Contains small amounts of three highly undesirable saturated fatty acids.
‡C10 to C16 indicate fatty acids with a chain length of 10 to 16 carbons, which are atherogenic.

TABLE 16.3

CEF Indexes of Red Meat
(for each 3.5-ounce or 100-gram edible portion)*

Beef		Heart	+4
Short rib (barbecued rib)	+31	Stew beef, lean	+4
Sirloin, choice	+24		
Whole rib (roast beef)	+22	*Pork*	
Brisket	+20	Spare ribs	+20
T-bone steak	+17	Pork chops	+17
Chuck pot roast	+17	Ham	+9
Regular hamburger	+17	Pork feet	+9
Tongue (untrimmed)	+17	Pork chops, lean	+8
Porterhouse	+16	Ham, lean	+4
Tenderloin	+12	*Lamb, Veal, Venison*	
Ground, lean	+12	Lamb chops, loin (2)	+42
Ground, extra lean	+10	Leg of lamb	+16
Round, eye or tip	+9	Leg of lamb, lean	+6
Corned beef	+9	Lamb chops, loin, lean (2)	+6
Liver	+8		
Kidneys	+6	Veal, lean	+6
Roundtop, tenderloin, lean meat	+5	Veal, leg	+6
		Venison	+4

*These CEF indexes are for only 100-gram (or ⅕-pound) portions. The total CEF index of a one-pound sirloin steak is +110.

TABLE 16.4

CEF Indexes of Seafood and Poultry
(for each 3.5-ounce or 100-gram edible portion)

Seafood, Fish, Frog Legs*

Squid	+2
King mackerel	0
Cod, dolphin, octopus	0
Bass, bluefish, catfish	−1
Croaker, flounder grouper, haddock, halibut	−1
Frog legs	−1
Perch, rockfish	−1
Shark, snapper, sole, swordfish	−1
Trout (rainbow or sea)	−1
Mackerel, Atlantic	−2
Salmon (Atlantic and coho)	−2
Tuna	−3
Trout, lake	−4

Shellfish

Lobster, shrimp	0
Snails	0
Oysters, scallops, crab, mussels	−1
Clams	−2

Poultry

Duck with skin (roasted)	+17
Chicken wings, fried	+10
Chicken, dark meat with skin (fried)	+9
Chicken, dark meat with skin (roasted)	+7
Duck without skin (roasted)	+6
Chicken liver	+6
Cornish hen, roasted	+5
Chicken, light meat with skin (fried)	+5
Turkey, dark meat with skin	+5
Chicken, light meat with skin (roasted)	+4
Pheasant, quail (roasted)	+4
Turkey, light meat with skin	+4
Turkey, dark meat without skin	+2
Chicken, dark meat without skin	+2
Turkey, light meat without skin	+1
Chicken, light meat without skin	+1
Turkey, sliced	+1

*The CEF Index of wild fish is slightly lower than that of farm-raised fish.

TABLE 16.5

CEF Indexes of Processed Meats
(for each 3.5-ounce or 100-gram edible portion,
unless otherwise indicated)

Bacon, fried (3 strips = +4)	+27	Ham and cheese roll (2 slices = +8)	+13
Bologna, beef or pork (2 slices = +14)	+22	Turkey hot dogs (1 frank = +6)	+12
Sausages, beef or pork (2 patties = +9) (2 links = +4)	+22	Turkey bologna (2 slices = +3)	+9
Hot dogs, beef or pork (1 frank = +11)	+22	Picnic loaf (pork and beef) (2 slices = +5)	+9
Pastrami (2 slices = +10)	+20	Corned beef (2 slices = +3)	+5
Salami and similar cold cuts (2 slices = +8)	+19	Chicken roll (2 slices = +2)	+4
Beef, lunch meat (2 slices = +10)	+18	Turkey roll (2 slices = +2)	+4
Ham patties (1 patty = +10)	+17	Turkey breast	+1

TABLE 16.6

CEF Indexes of Dairy Products, Eggs, Pasta, and Grains
(for each 3.5-ounce or 100-gram edible portion,
unless otherwise indicated)

Cream

Whipped   +45
(1 tbs = +6)

Whipped, light   +37
(1 tbs = +5)
(pressurized,
1 tbs = +1) .

Sour cream   +24
(1 tbs = +3)

Half-and-half   +14
(1 tbs = +2)

Cheeses

Cream cheese   +38

Cheddar   +38
(1 slice = +11)

American   +36
(1 slice = +9)

Colby, Gruyère,   +36
Muenster,
Roquefort
(1 slice = +9)

Provolone   +34
(1 slice = +9)

Parmesan   +34
(1 tbs, grated = +6)

Swiss   +31
(1 slice = +8)

Feta   +30

Mozzarella   +23
(1-oz slice = +7)

Mozzarella, part skim   +19

Cheez Whiz   +19

Ricotta, whole-milk   +14
(½ cup = +18)

Light (or Lite) Cheeses

American, Cheddar,   +13
Swiss
(1-oz slice = +4)

Ricotta, part skim   +10
(½ cup = +11)

Other Dairy Products

Cocoa   +21
(8-oz glass)

Eggnog (nonalcoholic)   +20
(8-oz glass)

Chocolate milk, whole   +10
(8-oz glass)

Milk shake   +9
(8-oz glass)

Whole milk   +9
(8-oz glass)

(cont'd)

CEF Indexes of Dairy Products, Eggs, Pasta, and Grains (*cont'd*)

Chocolate milk, 2% fat (8-oz glass)	+6	Sunny-side up (2 eggs + butter)	+18
Cottage cheese, creamed	+6	Hard-boiled or soft-boiled (2 eggs)	+10
Milk, 2% fat (8-oz glass)	+4		
Yogurt	+4	*Pasta and Grains*	
Yogurt, 2% fat	+2	Lasagna with meat and cheese	+10
Cottage cheese, 2% fat	+2	Macaroni and cheese, ravioli	+8
Fat-free milk, shakes, yogurt, or cottage cheese	0	Pancakes and waffles	+5
		Spaghetti with meat sauce	+3
		Plain pastas (without meat or cheeses)	+2
Eggs		Breads, rolls, buns (baked with milk and/or butter)	+2
Omelet with cheese	+22		
Egg yolk (1 medium = +5)	+21		
Omelet (2 eggs + butter)	+18	Plain rice (no butter or margarine added)	0

TABLE 16.7

CEF Indexes of Nuts, Fruits, and Vegetables
(for each 3.5-ounce or 100-gram edible portion)

Nuts		Peanuts, roasted	+3
Brazil, roasted	+9	Macadamia, roasted	0
Cashews, roasted	+6	Chestnuts	−1
Mixed nuts, roasted	+3	Pistachios	−5

CEF Indexes of Nuts, Fruits, and Vegetables (*cont'd*)

Filberts, roasted	−6
Almonds, roasted	−10
Pecans, walnuts	−11

Fruits

Coconut, dried (½-oz piece = +14)	+111
Coconut, dried flakes (⅛ cup = +16)	+62
Coconut, raw	+55
Coconut milk (juice) (½ cup = +55) (Coconut water, inside liquid = +1)	+40
Avocado	+3
Citrus fruits	0
All other fresh fruits, except figs	0
Dried fruits (apricots, peaches, cherries, dates, raisins, figs)	−1

Vegetables

French fries (5 pieces = +2)	+8
Hash browns (mashed potatoes = +2)	+8
Coleslaw	+4
Potato salad	+4
Soybeans	+1
Soybean curd (tofu)	+1
All other vegetables, including leaves, roots, stalks, or fruits (such as beans, cucumbers, corn, eggplant, peas [except chick-peas], peppers, pumpkin, squash, zucchini, tomatoes)	0
Chick-peas or garbanzo beans	−1
Herbs	−1

Cereal Products

Cheese crackers with peanut butter filling (5 pieces = +6)	+18
Ritz crackers (5 pieces = +2)	+14

(*cont'd*)

CEF Indexes of Nuts, Fruits, and Vegetables (*cont'd*)

Nacho chips (10 pieces = +2)	+11	Triscuit crackers (5 pieces = +2)	+7
Wheat Thins crackers (10 pieces = +2)	+9	Nearly all commercial cereals	−1
Graham crackers (5 pieces = +2)	+7		

TABLE 16.8

CEF Indexes of Frozen or Canned Foods

Sauces (*per 3.5 oz or 100 g*)

Béarnaise	+30
Tartar	+14
Hollandaise	+8
Spaghetti with meatballs	+3
Spaghetti with meat	+2
Spaghetti with tomato	+1
Marinara (tomato-based)	+1
Most other sauces without cheese, meat, or added oil	0

Soups (*per can*)

Cream of mushroom	+11
Chunky beef	+6
Minestrone	+4
Chicken noodle	+2
Clam chowder	+1
Most meatless soups	+1

Stuffings (*per 3.5 oz or 100 g*)

Stove Top: Chicken Florentine, vegetables with almond, garden herb, or wild rice with mushroom	+13
Other varieties	+9

Frozen Dinners (*per entrée*)

Salisbury steak, meat loaf, Swedish meatballs	+20
Enchiladas with beef and cheese (per 2 enchiladas)	+12

CEF Indexes of Frozen or Canned Foods (*cont'd*)

Most regular frozen dinners with red meat (Some with cheese or butter have higher CEF indexes.)	+10
Most regular frozen dinners w/chicken or turkey (Some in cream sauce, butter, or with cheese have much higher CEF indexes.)	+5

Most regular frozen dinners with seafoods (Some in cream sauce or butter have substantially higher CEF indexes.)	+4
Most Lite, Light, Lean, and Weight Watchers	+2
Most frozen pizzas are comparable to fresh pizzas (see Table 16.13)	

TABLE 16.9

CEF Indexes of Snacks and Desserts
(3.5-ounce or 100-gram portion)

Chocolate	+34	Cookies (made with butter)*	+15
Macaroons	+29	Chocolate icing	+14
Pound cake (made with butter)	+26	Cheese crackers	+13
Ice cream (17% fat)	+17	Cakes (made with butter)	+13
Chocolate chip cookies (made with butter)	+23	Chocolate-covered peanuts	+12
Chocolate-covered raisins (raisins + chocolate + milk + cocoa butter)	+18	Chocolate syrup	+12
		Hot chocolate (powder)	+10
Popcorn (butter added)	+17	Cakes with whipped cream and chocolate icing (and made with shortening)	+10
Brownies (made with butter)	+15		

(*cont'd*)

CEF Indexes of Snacks and Desserts (*cont'd*)

Most pastries (made with shortening)	+10	Plain cakes/cupcakes (made with shortening)	+6
Chocolate chip cookies (made with shortening)	+9	Light ice cream	+6
Chocolate fudge (made with shortening)	+9	Cookies (made with shortening)*	+5
Pound cakes (made with shortening)	+9	Blueberry muffins	+5
Caramel icing	+8	Butterscotch candies	+4
Chocolate fudge with nuts	+8	Most pies (apple, etc.)	+4
		Rice pudding	+4
Brownies (made with shortening)	+8	Tapioca pudding	+4
Eclairs with custard and chocolate icing	+6	Peanut brittle	+3
		Chocolate almonds	+3
Custard	+6	Fig bar	+1
Chocolate pudding	+6	Plain popcorn	+1
Peanut bar	+6	Pecan or walnut pie (baked with margarine)	+1
Doughnuts (plain)	+6	Sherbet, sorbet	0
		Frozen nonfat yogurt	0

*Butter cookies are generally 28–30 percent butter, so they will have a much higher CEF Index than other cookies.

TABLE 16.10

CEF Indexes of McDonald's Foods
(per serving unless otherwise indicated)

Breakfast

Biscuit with sausage and egg	+18
Sausage McMuffin with egg	+16
Biscuit with bacon, egg, and cheese	+15
Sausage McMuffin	+13
Biscuit with sausage	+13
Iced cheese danish	+9
Scrambled eggs	+8
Egg McMuffin	+8
Hot cakes with butter	+7
Pork sausage	+7
Hash-brown potatoes	+4
Cinnamon raisin danish	+4
Biscuit with spread	+4
English muffin with butter	+4
Apple/raspberry danish	+3

Big Mac	+15
Quarter Pounder	+14
Cheeseburger	+10
McLean Deluxe with cheese	+8
McLean Deluxe	+7
Chicken McNuggets	+7
Hamburger	+6
Filet-O-Fish	+6
McChicken	+6

Desserts

Chocolate chip cookies	+7
Apple pie	+7
Hot fudge sundae	+4
Vanilla cone or strawberry sundae (frozen yogurt)	+1
Low-fat shakes	+1
McDonaldland cookies	+1

Sandwiches

McRib	+22
Quarter Pounder with cheese	+19
McDLT	+18

Side Dishes

Chef salad*	+11
Garden salad	+6
French fries (large) (small = +3)	+5

*The CEF Index is lower when shredded carrots are substituted for cheese.

(cont'd)

CEF Indexes of McDonald's Foods (*cont'd*)

Chunky chicken or side salad	+2	Thousand island	+6
		Peppercorn	+5
		Ranch	+4
Salad Dressings (*per package*)		Lite vinaigrette, or reduced-calorie French	+1
Blue cheese	+8		

TABLE 16.11

CEF Indexes of Burger King Foods
(per serving unless otherwise indicated)

Breakfast		Bagel with bacon, egg, and cheese	+15
Danish	+40		
Scrambled egg platter with sausage	+23	Croissandwich with egg and cheese	+14
Bagel with sausage, egg, and cheese	+22	Bagel with ham, egg, and cheese	+13
Croissandwich with sausage, egg, and cheese	+22	Croissandwich with ham, egg, and cheese	+13
Scrambled egg platter with bacon	+19	Bagel with cream cheese	+13
Scrambled egg platter	+16	Biscuit with bacon and egg	+12
Biscuit with sausage and egg	+16	Biscuit with sausage	+11
Croissandwich with bacon, egg, and cheese	+15	Milk, whole	+11
		Bagel with egg and cheese	+10

CEF Indexes of Burger King Foods (*cont'd*)

Biscuit with bacon	+7	Cheeseburger	+14
French toast sticks	+5	Hamburger deluxe	+10
Hash browns or biscuit	+4	Chicken sandwich	+10
		Ocean Catch fish filet	+6
Bagel	+2	Chicken Tenders	+5
		Fish Tenders	+4

Sandwiches

Side Dishes

Double Whopper with cheese	+41	Chocolate, strawberry, or vanilla shake	+11
Double Whopper	+33		
Whopper with cheese	+28	Chef salad	+9
Bacon double cheeseburger deluxe	+27	Garden salad	+6
		Chunky chicken salad	+2
Bacon double cheeseburger	+26	Bleu cheese salad dressing	+7
Double cheeseburger	+24		
Mushroom double cheeseburger	+22	Thousand island salad dressing	+6
Whopper	+20	French dressing	+2
Cheeseburger deluxe	+15	French fries (small)	+2

TABLE 16.12

CEF Indexes of Hardee's Menu
(per serving unless otherwise indicated)

Breakfast

Big Country with sausage	+25
Big Country with country ham	+16
Big Country with bacon	+16
Canadian Rise 'N' Shine biscuit	+14
Bacon, egg, and cheese biscuit	+13
Steak and egg biscuit	+13
Sausage and egg biscuit	+12
Big Country breakfast (ham)	+12
Ham, egg, and cheese biscuit	+10
Three pancakes with sausage	+10
Sausage or steak biscuit	+9
Cinnamon 'N' Raisin	+8
Biscuit 'N' Gravy, or bacon and egg biscuit, or country ham with egg biscuit	+7
Ham and egg biscuit, or pancakes with bacon	+6
Bacon biscuit	+5
Chicken biscuit, or hash rounds	+4
Three pancakes, or country ham biscuit	+3
Rise 'N' Shine biscuit	+2

Salads

Chef salad	+18
Garden salad	+15
Chicken and pasta salad	+3

Sandwiches

Bacon cheeseburger	+27
Quarter pound cheeseburger	+26
Mushroom 'N' Swiss burger	+24
Big Deluxe burger	+21
Big Twin	+20
All-beef hot dog	+14
Cheeseburger	+13
Hot Ham 'N' Cheese	+11
Big Roast Beef	+10
Fisherman's Fillet	+8
Hamburger or regular roast beef	+8
Turkey Club	+7

CEF Indexes of Hardee's Menu (*cont'd*)

Chicken sticks (9 pieces)	+5	Cool Twist sundae (hot fudge)	+11
Chicken sticks (6 pieces)	+4		
Chicken Fillet and Crispy Curls	+4	Chocolate or strawberry shake	+9
Grilled chicken, or regular french fries	+2	Cool Twist sundae (caramel or strawberry)	+9
		Cool Twist cones	+7
Shakes and Desserts		Apple turnover or Big Cookie	+6
Vanilla shake	+12		

TABLE 16.13

CEF Indexes of Pizza Hut Pizza
(per 2 slices, medium size)

Hand-Tossed		***Thin 'N Crispy***	
Cheese	+28*	Super Supreme	+21
Supreme	+26	Pepperoni	+20
Super Supreme	+25	Supreme	+20
Pepperoni	+25	Cheese (or vegetarian)	+19
Pan Pizza		***Personal Pan Pizza*** (*whole*)	
Supreme	+25	Pepperoni	+20
Super Supreme	+21	Supreme	+18†
Pepperoni	+16		
Cheese (or vegetarian)	+16		

*68 percent of its fat is saturated.
†40 percent of its fat is saturated.

TABLE 16.4

CEF Indexes of Kentucky Fried Chicken
(one piece unless otherwise indicated)

Chicken Part	Extra Crispy	Original Recipe
Thigh	+11	+9
Breast	+8	+6
Chicken Nuggets (6)	—	+6
Drumstick	+5	+4

17

The CEF Index
Guidelines: A Flexible
Dietary Alternative

In the flexible dietary guidelines proposed here, there are no menus, recipes, or exchange lists. Choose a variety of foods with the lowest possible CEF indexes so that your total daily CEF Index of all foods and snacks does not exceed +30. Ideally, the total should remain under +20, but there is no need for panic if an occasional meal raises the daily CEF Index to +35 or +40, or if you are not sure about portion sizes and a precise CEF for a given meal. There should be no guilt over eating two eggs or a piece of beef from time to time. A single meal, a full day, or even an entire week of dietary indiscretion has no relevance to coronary heart disease. What counts is your long-term automatic recognition and selection of foods with low CEF indexes, while avoiding those with high indexes.

Practicality and Flexibility

It is essential to be practical and flexible in any long-term health promotion activity. The CEF Index discourages an isolated focus on a single nutrient such as saturated fat, cholesterol, or fish oil.

Instead, the cardiovascular impact of all major nutrients in foods is condensed into a single number. The CEF Index simplifies your task, avoiding information overload, confusion over how much of or what ingredients are present in a given food, and what they mean individually or collectively. It eliminates the need for a rigid diet, daily menus, food exchanges, itemized guidelines, and saturated fatty acid and cholesterol tables, and relieves the boredom, frustration, or anger over a lack of control or choice. The CEF Index also allows you to select from a variety of foods based on taste, habits, ethnic background, culture, and convenience. There are some restrictions on your choices, but so long as the CEF Index of all daily foods is under +30, you will be able to choose from a vast variety of foods.

Nutritional Misinformation

Food labels in the United States, which have long been inadequate, frequently give very little useful information to consumers. Many food packages designed to catch your attention in the supermarket create misconceptions by such claims as "no cholesterol," "100 percent pure vegetable oil," or "low sodium" while omitting other valuable information. Even when the Food and Drug Administration's new guidelines for nutritional labels are fully implemented, important information such as the levels of omega-3 or omega-6 polyunsaturates and trans fatty acids will not be made available to consumers.

Although all-purpose vegetable shortenings, baking and deep-frying fats, or stick margarines are "100 percent cholesterol-free" and "100 percent pure vegetable fats," they have approximately 25 percent saturated fatty acids. In addition, they have up to 30 percent trans fatty acids, which are even worse for the heart than saturated fats. From a cardiovascular perspective, these "pure" and "cholesterol-free" vegetable fats behave as if they have about 60 percent saturated fat, and their CEF indexes are even higher than those of beef tallow or lard. Contrary to commercials and labels, these are far from being "heart-friendly" or "heart-healthy" products.

Coconut and palm kernel oils are also "100 percent cholesterol-free" and "100 percent natural," but they have 92 percent and 82 percent SFA, respectively—and CEF indexes of +52 and +46 (for 2 tablespoons). These are more than twice the CEF of beef tallow or lard.

The term "vegetarian" is often associated with "heart-friendly" foods, but this is not always the case. For example, a vegetarian pizza from Pizza Hut and others has the same CEF Index as a regular cheese pizza—about +20 for two slices.

Seafood in a Flexible Diet

Seafood, including shellfish, is among the most desirable food items. All shellfish are extremely low in fat content (between 1.2 percent to 3.6 percent) and saturated fatty acids (less than 1 percent). In addition, because of their low energy density (fewer calories per 3.5-ounce portion), they are extremely suitable for overweight individuals and diabetics, even those with abnormal blood lipids. More important, seafood has a very high concentration of omega-3 polyunsaturated fats (up to 45 percent of their fat content). Table 8.1 (page 45) provides a summary of cholesterol and fatty acid composition of various fish and shellfish.

The exclusion of shellfish from many low-fat diets is based on old data, derived from obsolete chemical analyses. The reason for this exclusion is that shellfish contain small amounts of cholesterol as well as some cholesterol-like substances that are counted along with the cholesterol, even though they are not absorbed and are harmless. For example, each 3.5 ounces (100 grams) of oysters contain only 47 milligrams of cholesterol, but they also contain 75 milligrams of nonabsorbable cholesterol look-alikes. Clams have only 36 milligrams of cholesterol in each 3.5-ounce portion but also 120 milligrams of cholesterol look-alikes. In the past, chemical analyses measured both cholesterol and cholesterol-like substances; however, modern technology has enabled us to distinguish the difference between the two. What is almost always missing from discussions regarding shellfish is that cholesterol lookalikes actually reduce the absorption of dietary cholesterol and are therefore extremely beneficial.

The only shellfish with a relatively high cholesterol content is squid (280 milligrams per 3.5-ounce portion), but it is not very popular in the United States and is rarely consumed on a regular basis or in large quantitites. Shrimp is somewhere in the middle, with 157 milligrams of cholesterol in each 3.5-ounce portion. In fact, the cholesterol content of 10 ounces of shrimp is similar to that of only two eggs. However, because of shrimp's extremely low saturated fat content (.3 gram per 3.5 ounces) and its high concentration of desirable omega-3 polyunsaturates, it is still preferable to a variety of other foods.

The amount of cardioprotective omega-3 polyunsaturated fat varies in different fish, as well as in the same fish from various regions, depending on what the fish eats. More important, in the same fish the levels of omega-3 polyunsaturates may be 2–3 times higher in wild, as compared to farm-raised, fish.

The problem is not the seafood but how it is prepared. Obviously, drowning it in butter or a creamy sauce defeats the purpose. No formula, CEF Index or otherwise, can predict how much butter or cream the cook may add to a given serving of seafood, or to any other food. It is therefore essential both at home and away from home to avoid foods prepared with ingredients that have a high CEF Index (+34 for butter versus +1 for olive oil, per 2 tablespoons).

Meat in a Flexible Diet

Nearly all low-fat meats, including chicken and turkey, veal, and lean beef, have very low concentrations of total and saturated fats and relatively low cholesterol. Lean cuts of beef do not raise the blood cholesterol level any more than do chicken or fish. Recent studies have demonstrated that it is beef fat, not the beef itself, that raises the levels of LDL cholesterol in the blood. If you shop for beef that is not marbled, lean beef can be included in a cholesterol-lowering diet. Use of lean cuts of beef and pork, or beef and chicken hearts (CEF Index +4), may allow for more flexibility and palatability in the diet.

Brains have a very high cholesterol content–nearly 1,800 milligrams per 3.5-ounce portion, an amount equivalent to the cholesterol present in eight eggs! Clearly it is best to avoid this item. Liver, kidneys, and sweetbreads (pancreas) have a very low fat content of approximately 3 percent but a cholesterol content of approximately 300 to 400 milligrams per 3.5 ounces. Because of their very low fat content, and especially their extremely low SFA, their CEF indexes are not high (+6 for kidneys and +8 for beef liver). For this reason, they could be occasional choices in a flexible dietary program, provided they are not fried, served with butter sauces, or consumed in large portions (more than 3.5 ounces).

Vegetables, Fruit, and Grains in a Flexible Diet

Vegetables, fruits, and grains, once an afterthought in the diet, were treated as third- or fourth-class nutrients. A piece of fruit, butter-coated vegetables, or sprigs of parsley traditionally adorned dishes overflowing with béarnaise or hollandaise sauce. Grains and legumes have struggled for respectability (and edibility). Meats and fats therefore held center stage in most meals. In the United States, on any given day, 50 percent of adults eat no garden vegetables, and more than 40 percent eat no fruits. Although the 1990 dietary recommendations of the Nutrition Board of the National Academy of Sciences call for five or more servings of vegetables and fruits, at least 35 percent of the U.S. adults on average eat only two (or fewer) servings per day.

Vegetables, fruits, and grains are first-class nutrients for cardiovascular health. Because of their very low CEF indexes, their ability to satisfy hunger without a lot of extra calories, and the potential to displace saturated fats (by substituting for "rich" foods), they provide some of the most desirable and "heart-friendly" foods in a flexible diet. Just as important is their abundance of various essential minerals, vitamins, antioxidants, and other nutrients.

Total CEF Index of Foods

Because the CEF Index is not a quantitative, mathematical, or bio-chemical score, it cannot be assumed that consuming foods with a low CEF Index will entirely counteract or neutralize the effects of foods with a high CEF Index. In fact, as emphasized for fish and shellfish, the beneficial effect of some foods may be lost or sub-stantially diluted if ingredients with very high CEF indexes (e.g., butter, cream, and cheese) are added to nutrients with low indexes.

The CEF Index was developed to allow variety, choice, and flex-ibility in eating. Therefore, you will defeat its purpose if you con-sume too much of any one food group—especially one with high CEF indexes—and ignore others.

The total or final CEF Index of all foods is obviously dependent on the portion size. Although the CEF Index of a 3.5-ounce piece of lean beef (lean top round or tenderloin) is +9, the CEF Index of a 10-ounce tenderloin steak is +27. For this reason, the quan-tity of foods is an independent but inseparable factor that must be considered in any dietary program, especially for overweight or diabetic individuals.

18

Recommendations for a Flexible Diet

The CEF Index offers a simple and accessible way to know the cardiovascular effects of hundreds of foods. However, as with most scoring systems, there are some cautions. To improve the effectiveness of the CEF Index, keep the following guidelines in mind:

- *The ideal daily CEF Index is under +20.* Nevertheless, ideal things are often impractical, and there is plenty of room for flexibility, provided your total daily CEF Index does not exceed +30. Try to keep the CEF Index of at least one meal (breakfast or lunch) under +5.
- *Use the CEF Index for all your grocery shopping.* This is especially useful when selecting meats, oils, and processed foods. The CEF Index should reduce the misleading role of deceptive advertising or unclear information on food labels.
- *Marbled red meat is a major culprit, with a high CEF Index.* For this reason, trim off visible fat before and after cooking. Sometimes the fat is inseparable from the meat.

Forget about barbecued ribs, since they aren't worth their high CEF Index of +31 for a 3.5-ounce portion. Instead, buy extra-lean ground beef, seafood, or poultry. To see how trimming the fat dramatically alters the CEF Index, look at lamb chops and pork chops in Table 16.3. The CEF Index for two lamb chops is +42, whereas the CEF Index for the lean meat of the same chops is only +6. The respective indexes for regular and trimmed pork chops are +17 and +8.

Most of us are not sure of the fat content of various meats, nor do we eat extremely lean red meats. As shown in Table 16.3, most red meats have relatively high CEF indexes. To avoid eating a meal with a very high CEF Index, keep the portion size of practically all red meats under 7 to 8 ounces—and preferably around 3.5 to 4 ounces.

It is a common misunderstanding that poultry should be skinned before cooking. Baking, broiling, or grilling chicken or turkey with skin does not transfer the fat to the meat. Skinning poultry before cooking can turn it into a tough or juiceless meat. Leave the skin on when cooking, but don't eat it once the meat is done.

• *Eat seafood at least three to four times a week.* This also cuts down the number of times you eat other fatty meals. Any seafood or shellfish is superior to all other meats, provided it is not cooked with butter, margarine, or vegetable shortening and is not covered with cheese or cream sauces. Large amounts of omega-6 PUFA present in vegetable oils and fats will block the entry of beneficial seafood omega-3 fatty acids into various cells, including platelets. As noted in chapter 8, platelets with high concentrations of omega-6 PUFA can cause intravascular clotting, quite the opposite of platelets containing omega-3.

Eating seafood frequently is one of the most effective ways of cutting down the risk of heart attack. You can have a tuna sandwich (no mayonnaise or butter) for lunch two days a week, then have two seafood dinners in between when fresh seafood can be purchased or when you eat out.

• *Big portions almost always mean not only more calories but also higher CEF indexes.* There is no incentive for stores to sell a small piece of meat when a larger piece is more profitable. Just because the steak comes in a large size, it doesn't mean it should all be eaten in one sitting. Share the large piece, or cut it in half for another meal. Overeating and caloric excess are nutritional sins we pay for in high rates of obesity, diabetes, atherosclerosis, and various cancers. The parental encouragement (or command) to "clean your plate" was for growing up; there is no need to keep that commandment now that we are adults.

• *Avoid "all-you-can-eat," "smorgasbord," "buffet," or "two-for-one" meals.* Such promotions are traps where sight and smell overwhelm good judgment. When entrapped, choose more vegetables, fruits, salads, lean meats, and starchy items such as rice, potatoes, and breads (but no butter or cheese).

• *Substitute canola or olive oil for butter, cream, margarine, or vegetable shortening.* Just because a recipe recommends butter, you don't have to follow it exactly. Compromise in favor of your heart, not the recipe.

• *Avoid or cut down deep-frying and the use of all-purpose vegetable shortening or stick margarine.* It is a dietary misconception to assume that we can safely substitute these fats for butter, and there are 10 reasons why they are not as safe as advertised (see chapter 8). Potato chips and corn chips have as much as 35 percent fat, and about one-third of this fat is atherogenic trans fatty acids. Even most ready-to-eat or microwave popcorns have 25 percent fat with one-third trans fatty acids. Creamy peanut butter is also a processed fatty product, with variable amounts of undesirable saturated and trans fatty acids. The less animal fat or processed vegetable fat in the diet, the better.

• *Experiment with the amount of oil or fat called for in a recipe.* Regardless of what the recipe says, reduce the oil by one-half or one-third—and even then, use canola or olive oil. If you can't use canola or olive oil, use small amounts of light canola margarine in place of melted butter or vegetable shortening.

• *Avoid cream, cheese, or butter-based sauces.* In restaurants, ask your server directly how a given sauce is prepared. Choose a dish with no cream or butter sauce, or ask for "only a touch" of the sauce on the side. (The CEF Index of béarnaise sauce is +9 for 2 tablespoons, and that does not include the rest of the meal.) Many Italian sauces have a tomato base (with or without olive oil) and are more reasonable choices, but again, pay attention to the quantity.

• *Use herbs, spices, and vegetables in your cooking.* Certain vegetables and all green vegetables, such as broccoli, brussels sprouts, cabbage, cauliflower, kale, leeks, romaine or butterhead lettuce, and spinach, and green herbs such as basil, marjoram, oregano, and parsley are extremely low in fat (less than 1 percent). However, a large portion of this fat is the desirable omega-3 polyunsaturate variety. More important, these vegetables and herbs add flavor and personality to food. All sauces without meat, cheese, or added fat have very low CEF indexes and are therefore terrific for adding zest and flavor without the calories and the high CEF Index of various fats.

• *Make your own salad dressing with olive oil or canola oil.* You can also dilute the oil with water or wine, or use the "lite" or low-calorie variety. Most regular commercial salad dressings are 50 to 70 percent fat and more than 12 to 14 percent saturated fat. Many, such as blue cheese, thousand island, and French, contain cottonseed oil—with a very high CEF Index.

• *Switch to low-fat or skim milk.* Several reports have suggested a weak association between consumption of whole milk or whole-milk products and coronary heart disease. Although milk's fat may well be part of the problem, there is also an enzyme in whole milk, xanthine oxidase, that is a potent oxidant and may contribute to the oxidation of the "bad" LDL cholesterol into the "mean" LDL cholesterol. Even though the case against whole milk is far from proven, 1 or 2 percent milk is just as "wholesome" and nutritious as whole milk, and it has no adverse cardiovascular effect.

Except for cottage cheese, many cheeses are over 30 percent fat, with CEF indexes of +45 or higher. Even ricotta or light mozzarella has a fat content of 14 to 20 percent. Two slices of cheddar or American cheese have a CEF Index of +22 and +18, respectively. Dairy foods are one area where flexibility and freedom of choice should be balanced for health.

• *Many processed meats (sausages, hot dogs, salami, or bologna) have CEF indexes in excess of +20.* Even worse would be a sandwich such as bologna and cheese with mayonnaise or butter. On the other hand, processed ham, turkey, chicken, or lean beef are reasonable choices. Note, too, that an occasional hot dog, submarine sandwich, two strips of bacon, or two links of sausage won't choke off anyone's coronary arteries.

• *In fast-food restaurants, avoid deep-fried dishes and those made with cheese.* Look at CEF indexes for various fast foods in tables 16.9 through 16.13. Choose among fast foods with low CEF indexes (see Chapter 19).

• *Do not deep-fry foods that have a low CEF Index.* Cooking chicken, turkey, lean red meats, and seafood in shortening, butter, or margarine is self-defeating. After all, your oven has settings for baking, broiling, or grilling, so the addition of oil is not necessary. To sauté, use a nonstick pan and a vegetable oil spray, olive oil, or canola oil.

• *Cheesecake, pastries, and cookies invariably have very high CEF indexes.* Substitute sherbet, fruit, simple cake, or even pecan pie (pecans have 8 to 10 percent of the "heart-friendly" omega-3 polyunsaturates) or low-fat fruit pie. Low-fat or nonfat frozen yogurt has a CEF Index of $+0$ to $+2$. Table 16.9 provides a number of other reasonable desserts to choose from, including some made with chocolate. Also keep in mind the portion of the dessert. (The CEF Index for a *pound* of "light" ice cream is $+30$ and for brownies $+40$, in case of temptation!)

• *Be skeptical of food labels.* The label on a popular nondairy coffee creamer clearly states that it "may contain" coconut, palm, palm kernel, and cottonseed oils. All four ingredients have extremely high CEF indexes (Table 16.2). Occasional use of this or any other product with a very high CEF Index is probably not relevant to cardiovascular events, but frequent (several times a day) and long-term use of such products is unwise. This also holds true for hydrogenated vegetable oils such as stick margarine or shortening, which contain a high concentration of saturated and trans fatty acids.

• *The percentage of fat in foods is a useless figure.* The percentage of *calories from fat*, however, is meaningful. Food packages that proclaim in large print "only 25 percent fat" are referring to percent by weight, not by calories. For example, beef or pork hot dogs contain about 35 percent fat by weight, but approximately 80 percent of their calories come from fat. Turkey and chicken hot dogs are only slightly better, with approximately 70 percent of their calories coming from fat. Natural hard cheeses are 30 percent fat by weight, with 70 percent of their calories coming from fat. For potato chips or corn chips, over 50 percent of calories come from fat.

Even in a large serving of fish, only about 10 percent of the calories come from fat. If the same fish is covered with butter or cream sauces, up to 70 percent of the calories may come from fat, and its CEF Index of about $+1$ may go up to $+10$. As a practical rule, a meal should derive no more than 30 percent of its calories from fat. When in doubt, use the CEF Index.

• *Do not skip meals.* Many overweight people mistakenly assume that eating one meal must be better than eating three. Numerous studies in both laboratory animals and human volunteers have shown that fewer meals often result in more efficient absorption and metabolism of nutrients. All of this contributes to weight gain. Recent studies have also shown that when people eat one to two meals per day, they have higher levels of the "bad" LDL cholesterol than when they eat three to four smaller meals per day. This is true even if their intake of fats and calories is reduced. The scientific explanation for this is that we release a higher amount of insulin into our blood in response to fewer and bigger meals. High levels of blood insulin increase the levels of both LDL and VLDL cholesterol. The activity of LDL receptors in the liver is also reduced during many hours of not eating, so the LDL particles are not grabbed by these receptors for disposal. So eat three or four smaller meals per day.

• *Don't use vacations or holidays for overindulgence.* If we use the CEF Index on these occasions (and we should at all times), they needn't be blamed for our downfall.

19

Fast Foods and the Heart

❦

Nearly one-half of the respondents in a recent survey said they eat at a fast-food restaurant at least once a week, and 22 percent said they do so every day or several times a week. However, 54 percent of those interviewed acknowledged that fast foods are "not too good" or "not good at all."

The Appeal of Fast Foods

The reason so many people eat fast foods even though they question the nutritional quality is that such foods are fast, safe (at least for the short term), consistently prepared, familiar, and convenient, and provide cost-effective meals. All fast foods are not "junk foods." Many are healthful, nutritious, tasty, and affordable. The problem is that consumers often do not exercise their options or choose among many reasonable and nutritious meals available at fast-food establishments.

All Fast Foods Are Not the Same

Hamburgers, cheeseburgers, salads, and pizzas can vary from one fast-food establishment to the next. In tables 16.10 to 16.13, CEF indexes of comparable foods at various chain restaurants are different. Of course, you can always stay away from all restaurants

serving foods with high CEF indexes, since options are more limited there. But at a fast-food eatery like Burger King, you are certainly not forced to order a Double Whopper with cheese (with a
very high CEF Index of +41) and a chocolate shake (CEF Index
of +11). You could order instead the Ocean Catch Fish Filet
(+5), Chicken Tenders (+5), Fish Tenders (+3), or Chunky
Chicken Salad (+2).

The CEF Indexes of Fast Foods

The size of a fast-food meal determines its total CEF Index. For
example, the CEF Index of one single slice of medium-size, hand-
tossed cheese pizza from Pizza Hut is +14. But the pizza industry
would not sell $22 billion worth of pizza every year if most people
ate only one slice. So by the time you have finished three slices,
containing over 900 milligrams of salt and 30 grams of fat (68 percent of which is saturated), you have devoured a CEF Index of
+42. If you crave pizza, avoid meat pizzas and those with extra
cheese. Ask for less cheese and less meat but more vegetables.

Recently "vegetarian" pizzas have been promoted as being
healthful. A vegetarian pizza (Pizza Hut and others) is just a cheese
pizza with vegetables on top, carrying a heavy and undesirable
CEF Index of approximately +30 for three slices.

Fast-food chains have tried to improve their nutritional image.
More salads and fewer fatty foods adorn their new menus. Lean
deluxe ground beef, vegetable oil for french fries, 1 percent milk,
breakfast cereal, and shredded carrots instead of cheese on salads
are all steps in the right direction. Recently some of the fast food
chains such as McDonald's have unfortunately regressed by adding very high CEF Index foods (i.e., Double Quarter Pounder with
Cheese and McRib) to their menus or are test marketing other
heart-unfriendly menus.

Good intentions or otherwise, fast-food eateries also have to sell
their products, and they cannot sell good nutrition when the food
does not look or taste good. Unfortunately, this becomes a catch-
22 in the marketing of these foods, including "healthy" salads.

Salads are commonly associated with good nutrition. In most

fast-food restaurants, however, various cheeses, meats, and hard-boiled eggs, not to mention dressings, are added, dramatically changing their CEF indexes. The CEF Index of Burger King's or McDonald's Chunky Chicken Salad is only +2, which is excellent. On the other hand, the chef and garden salads at Hardee's score +18 and +15, at McDonald's +11 and +6, and at Burger King +9 and +6, respectively. By the time dressing is added, salads are not as healthful as advertised. Even the most nutritionally conscientious consumer wouldn't imagine that a salad could be worse than a cheeseburger, a hot dog, or a big roast beef sandwich.

Another example of good intentions gone awry are the baked potatoes at Wendy's and other fast-food restaurants. A plain baked potato is a good and healthful food with a CEF Index of 0, but when stuffed with cheese, bacon, and melted margarine, it is converted into a meal with a CEF Index of +15. Suggestion: Ask for no added oil, half the cheese, and only a touch of bacon.

How to Choose a Meal at a Fast-Food Restaurant

It is estimated that nearly 50 percent of all meals in the United States are eaten away from home. From a health perspective, eating at a fast-food restaurant is really no different from eating at any other establishment.

Various hamburgers, cheeseburgers, and fried chicken are the backbone of many fast-food eateries, but the size, shape, garnishes, and other additions (bacon, fried onions, or mushrooms, etc.) can change the CEF Index of a hamburger or chicken sandwich in a fast-food place. No one expects you to carry around CEF indexes for every hamburger or salad you may ever run into. What is required is to have some understanding of the CEF indexes of basic menus served at these restaurants, as shown in tables 16.10 through 16.13. The scores may vary markedly for items with high CEF indexes, but those with indexes in the midrange or low range (simple burgers and roast beef, chicken, or fish sandwiches) are within a few points of one another.

No matter how a piece of chicken or fish is prepared, it inherently has a lot less saturated fat than ground beef; you are therefore better off choosing among these items. Peeling off the battered skin of fried chicken is easy, and quickly lowers the CEF Index of the meal by several points. Hardee's grilled chicken sandwich is very heart-healthy and nutritious, with a remarkably low CEF Index of +2. You can also choose a regular roast beef sandwich or hamburger there (CEF indexes of +8). But avoid the bacon cheeseburger (CEF Index +27) or quarter pound cheeseburger (CEF Index +26). At Burger King, a Double Whopper with cheese has a CEF Index of +41 and a regular Whopper with cheese has a CEF Index of +28. At McDonald's, a Quarter Pounder with cheese has a CEF Index of +19 and the McDLT has a CEF index of +18.

Double this or double that; "deluxe" burgers; and added items such as bacon, fried onions or mushrooms, mayonnaise, sauces, and various cheeses all raise the CEF Index. For breakfast, avoid the platters, sausages or bacon-and-cheese combinations—especially those with butter.

If you don't eat anything greasy at home, why do it away from home? You can exercise your options and be more selective wherever you eat.

20

Dietary and Life-Style Changes for Abnormal Blood Cholesterol

For decades, dietary interventions to improve cardiovascular health have focused exclusively on efforts to lower cholesterol levels. As explained previously, this is a narrow and limited aim, since only about 20 to 30 percent of persons with coronary heart disease have elevated levels of cholesterol. Dietary interventions should also raise the low levels of HDL cholesterol and address other modifiable risk factors, especially the potential to form blood clots (thrombosis) within coronary and cerebral arteries. It is disheartening that most current dietary interventions to lower blood cholesterol tend to reduce the "good" HDL cholesterol and lack an anti-thrombogenic effect. A dietary program based on the CEF Index avoids these pitfalls.

Lowering the "Bad" LDL Cholesterol

If a person's total cholesterol level is below 240 mg/dl (or the LDL cholesterol is under 160 mg/dl), and there are no other major risk

121

TABLE 20.1

Selective Intervention for Elevated LDL Cholesterol

LDL Cholesterol (mg/dl)	No Other Risk Factors*	Other Risk Factors Present
1. 130–160	• Maintain daily CEF Index of about +30. • Increase seafood consumption to three to four meals per week. • Exercise. • Normalize weight. • Add vitamin E at doses up to 800 to 1,000 mg daily.	• Maintain daily CEF Index of about +20 to +30. • Increase seafood consumption to three to four meals per week. • Treat other risk factors; exercise. • Add vitamin E (up to 800–1,000 mg/day). • If no response after six months, add appropriate cholesterol-lowering drugs (prescribed by physician).
2. 160–190	• Same as #1 above • If no response in six months, lower the daily CEF Index to about +20 to +30, and *consider* cholesterol-lowering drugs.	• Same as #1 above
3. High-risk levels (over 190)	• Same as #2 above. • Add appropriate cholesterol-lowering drugs if no response in six months (or in case	• Same as #1 above, *especially after coronary bypass surgery or angioplasty.*

Selective Intervention for Elevated LDL Cholesterol

LDL Cholesterol (mg/dl)	*No Other Risk Factors**	*Other Risk Factors Present*
	of poor compliance with above), especially in those under age 60–65.	• Add appropriate cholesterol-lowering drugs (prescribed by physician) promptly.

*Excluding age and gender
For CEF Index of various foods, see tables 16.1 through 16.14.

factors (excluding age and gender), there is no evidence that lowering blood cholesterol increases life expectancy or offers any significant cardiovascular benefit. Making life difficult for millions of people by imposing a rigid dietary program serves no purpose. Instead, a diet based on a total daily CEF Index of about +30 is reasonable and practical.

On the other hand, when elevated cholesterol levels are associated with other risk factors, the probability of cardiovascular events increases dramatically. Here it is inarguable that we should modify or treat as many risk factors as possible. For these individuals, any abnormal cholesterol level is undesirable, and a more disciplined approach for controlling risk factors is necessary (see Table 20.1).

People with coronary heart disease, especially at a young age, have more than an 80 percent chance of dying from cardiovascular events unless we intervene aggressively. They are the prime candidates for comprehensive risk reduction. A similar plan should be pursued in apparently healthy individuals if they have "high" blood cholesterol levels *and* a close family member who was diagnosed with CHD at a young age.

Raising the "Good" HDL Cholesterol

Contrary to current recommendations, a marked reduction of total dietary fat is difficult, counterproductive, and, when combined with a high intake of carbohydrates, may in fact reduce the blood level of the "good" HDL cholesterol by over 30 percent. The use of monounsaturated fats such as canola or olive oil in place of butter, lard, vegetable shortening, or margarines, along with a daily CEF Index of about +20 to +30, is the logical alternative.

Eating seafood, including shellfish, at least three or four times a week is one of the most cardioprotective dietary measures. Seafood also raises the blood level of the "good" HDL while lowering the "bad" VLDL and the two "mean" lipoproteins (see chapter 8).

Dry roasted nuts such as almonds, pistachios, pecans, or walnuts (but *not* peanuts or cashews), which have very desirable CEF indexes, are suitable snacks, unless you have a weight problem. Their fatty acids are primarily monounsaturated, but they also contain 6–10 percent omega-3 polyunsaturated fatty acids, which are "heart-friendly."

Vegetables, fruits, and herbs, especially as a component of weight-reducing programs, not only help lower the LDL but also increase the "good" HDL cholesterol.

Frequent but sensible exercise, whether accompanied by weight loss or as a component of a conditioning program, helps to increase the "good" HDL cholesterol. The type of exercise is less important than how regular and vigorous it is. At present, there are two ongoing studies dealing with the effects of leisure-time exercises and the reduced rates of CHD (one is in London, England, with civil service workers, and the other is in the United States, with Harvard University alumni; each one includes nearly 17,000 individuals). In both studies the risk of CHD seems to have been reduced approximately 50 percent by certain levels of exercise. A 17-year follow-up study of 5,000 Danish men in 1992 showed that low physical activity and a sedentary life-style were associated with a 70 percent increased risk of premature death from CHD, compared to those who engaged in a high level of leisure-time physical activity.

In this Danish report, and in many others, work-site physical work was not found to have a cardioprotective benefit. In addition, walking at work is practically never vigorous or steady enough to be useful. Routine walking up and down stairs (at home or at work) does not seem to be enough to reduce the risk of CHD. Jogging, fast-paced walking, biking, rowing, swimming, aerobic exercise and dance, cross-country skiing (open air or on machines), handball or racquetball, and body conditioning or bodybuilding are all exercises that may help to increase the HDL cholesterol. Playing a friendly game of doubles or even a leisurely singles game has too many interruptions and pauses to serve this purpose.

How often and how much exercise is needed for beneficial cardiovascular effects is not precise or fixed for all ages. Studies show that enough exercise to increase one's heart rate to 60 to 85 percent of the maximum for about 30 to 40 minutes, three or four times a week, is a good, attainable level for most people. Maximum heart rate equals 220 minus your age. For example, a 45-year-old person would have a maximum heart rate of $220 - 45 = 175$. Any exercise that sustains the heart rate between 105 and 146 beats per minute (60 to 85 percent of the maximum rate) for 30 to 40 minutes provides cardiovascular benefits. This level of exercise should be reached gradually, over days or weeks. However, individuals with even the slightest hint of CHD should not start any vigorous exercise program without their physician's evaluation and recommendation.

Regular exercise improves the heart's pumping action and in the long run lowers blood pressure by relaxing peripheral vessels and resistance to blood flow through the arteries. Exercise not only increases the production of the "good" HDL cholesterol, especially the cardioprotective HLD-2, but also reduces its breakdown in the bloodstream. In addition, fats entering the blood after meals are cleared away at a much faster pace in active people than in those who are sedentary. This is a significant bonus; delayed clearance of fats from the blood may be an important risk factor for coronary artery disease. Regular exercise may also promote a healthy life-style (such as not smoking, weight control, etc.) and reduce resistance to insulin and the risk of developing diabetes. Moreover, active people have lower mortality rates not only from coronary heart disease but also from cancer and other causes.

Smoking has many harmful effects. Many studies have shown that smoking more than doubles the risk of developing coronary heart disease. In one study, the mortality from CHD in those smoking 25 or more cigarettes per day was nearly triple that of nonsmokers. In women under the age of 55, smoking accounts for almost half of all heart attacks. Contrary to an almost universal misconception, smoking "low-tar" cigarettes does not appear to reduce these risks. Overall, in the United States alone, smoking is directly responsible for about 115,000 deaths from coronary heart disease each year (and a total death toll of over 470,000 a year).

Smoking increases the risk of coronary heart disease in several ways. It damages the inner wall of the arteries, increases the blood level of fibrinogen (a potent clotting factor), activates the blood platelets to release additional clotting factors into the blood, and causes spasm and constriction of coronary arteries, all of which may contribute to clogging of the arteries. Moreover, smoking reduces the HDL cholesterol by 10 to 20 percent in regular smokers. Quitting the habit results in a dramatic 50 to 70 percent reduction in the risk of heart attacks.

Losing weight by dieting alone, even if the weight loss is substantial, does not lower the "bad" LDL cholesterol or increase the "good" HDL cholesterol adequately, unless it is combined with regular exercise. During exercise, circulating blood fats and lipoproteins are broken down (metabolized), producing various byproducts including HDL cholesterol. Some dietary fat is necessary to promote this process, since it provides muscles with the ingredients they need to produce some HDL. This is another reason why very-low-fat diets are counterproductive in those with low HDL blood levels.

Weight "cycling," repeated cycles of losing weight and regaining it, may increase blood lipid abnormalities and the risk of coronary heart disease.

Alcohol in small to moderate amounts (less than three cocktails, three beers, or three glasses of wine per day) may reduce the risk of coronary artery disease, at least in part by raising the level of the cardioprotective HDL cholesterol. However, don't take up drinking just to "cleanse" your arteries. If you enjoy a couple of drinks with your dinner, there is no evidence to suggest any harm to your heart, and there might even be a small cardioprotective benefit. However, excessive drinking, even on occasion, has a vast number of side effects, easily overwhelming any conceivable cardiovascular benefit. (See chapter 14.)

Lowering VLDL and Triglyceride Levels

As noted in chapter 3, recent data strongly suggest that elevated triglycerides (and VLDL) are almost always associated with low levels of HDL, creating a more cardiovascular unfriendly environment. To cope with this problem, all the measures recommended here for raising HDL are equally relevant. For the high triglyceride levels, more emphasis must be placed on reducing total calories, specifically on reducing simple carbohydrates (sugars) as well as certain complex carbohydrates (such as white bread or pasta, potatoes, and white rice). All of these carbohydrates result in higher insulin and triglyceride levels. Weight loss accompanied by exercise and correction of other disorders such as diabetes, kidney or thyroid problems, and excessive alcohol intake should be considered first before using triglyceride-lowering drugs. Seafood and monounsaturated fats (such as olive oil) are actually good substitutes for high carbohydrate diets. Vegetable oils (omega-6 PUFA) are also counterproductive here. Overall, a daily CEF Index of between $+20$ and $+30$ provides a sensible dietary guideline.

What If Dietary and Life-Style Changes Fail to Improve Lipid Disorders?

Although coronary heart disease is the result of exposure to a variety of risk factors over many years, eliminating or modifying even a single risk factor can be enormously helpful (see Table 20.2). For example, the risk of having a coronary event for a middle-aged man who smokes, has high blood pressure, and shows a high level of blood cholesterol is about 21 per 1,000 per year. However, the risk for a nonsmoker with desirable blood pressure and normal blood cholesterol drops to about 2 per 1,000 per year. This is a dramatic 1,000 percent risk reduction. Of course, the relative

TABLE 20.2

Estimated Risk Reduction of Heart Attacks, by Type of Intervention

Intervention	Risk Reduction
Smoking cessation	50–70%
Lowering the LDL cholesterol	2% for every 1-mg/dl decline in LDL
Raising the HDL cholesterol	4% for every 1-mg/dl rise in HDL
Lowering the diastolic blood pressure	2% for every 1-mm/Hg decline
Exercise and active life-style	35–55%
Maintaining normal weight	35–55%
Alcohol (two to three drinks per day)	25–45%
Estrogen-replacement therapy	45%
Low doses of aspirin	30–35%
CEF Index of +20 to +30 per day	50%
Vitamin E (800–1,000 mg per day)	20%

impact or the estimated benefits vary from individual to individual. But it is important to aggresively modify as many risk factors as possible.

The measures recommended in this chapter, including adherence to a dietary program with a daily CEF Index at or below +30, should help to reduce the risk of coronary heart disease and its progression (if it has already occurred). For those who continue to have high-risk LDL or HDL levels, especially when other risk factors are also present, judicious and monitored addition of cholesterol-altering drugs may be justified. Here, the prime candidates for drug therapy are those with multiple risk factors and severe abnormalities in their blood lipids, younger persons with coronary heart disease, and persons with a close family member who developed CHD at a young age.

People who have already had coronary angioplasty (dilating the inside of blocked coronary arteries) or coronary bypass surgery are in a very-high-risk category. For them, the possibility that dilated coronary arteries or newly transplanted grafts will be reclogged is a major concern, especially for individuals with abnormal blood lipids. They do not have the luxury of time to wait and see if they respond to dietary and life-style changes. A vigorous program of total risk reduction is essential, both before and after surgery. Moreover, these persons must be started on cholesterol-altering drugs and a flexible dietary program with a CEF Index of less than +30. Although the role of antioxidants, including vitamin E, in the process of atherosclerosis and reclogging of the arteries is still far from proven, vitamin E at doses up to 800 to 1,000 milligrams per day is entirely safe and may indeed have a cardioprotective role. A significant increase in the consumption of seafood, which contains omega-3 polyunsaturates, should precede balloon angioplasty or coronary bypass surgery by at least several weeks and should continue indefinitely. Small doses of aspirin (80 to 100 milligrams per day) may further reduce the risk of a future coronary event—if your physician approves of such a regimen.

21

Nutritional Intervention
in the Older Population

At present, 1 percent of older Americans *below* the age of 75 and 20 percent of those *over* the age of 85 live in nursing homes. Many more require temporary stays in these facilities. Half of all individuals are in nursing homes because of chronic conditions that do not have specific risk factors. Of those not institutionalized, many suffer from various chronic diseases that require treatment. As the population ages, the prevalence of cardiovascular diseases, arthritis, and Alzheimer's will increase unless preventive measures are adopted. Unfortunately, for many of these chronic diseases (e.g., Alzheimer's) we currently have no effective prevention. Recent studies have shown that certain genetic abnormalities may predispose some people to develop these "degenerative" diseases. It may be years before the results of these studies can be applied to disease prevention or treatment. Today, however, we may be able to alter the occurrence of cardiovascular events, including angina, heart attack, stroke, cardiovascular disability, or death. To achieve this goal, we must intervene before coronary heart disease has set in or resulted in irreversible complications.

The Significance of Abnormal Blood Cholesterol in an Older Person

Elevated cholesterol levels are common in the elderly population. Twenty-four million Americans (one-third of men and one-half of women) over age 55 have blood cholesterol levels in excess of 240 mg/dl. But it is a myth that atherosclerosis and coronary heart disease are inevitable consequences of normal aging. They are not. Rather, they are the result of long-standing exposure to various risk factors, including abnormalities in certain blood lipids. Atherosclerosis is an ongoing process that worsens with aging. The progression of arterial injury, especially in coronary and brain arteries, explains the very high rates of heart attack and stroke in the older population. Much of this is preventable.

The death rate from CHD has shown a progressive decline over the past 40 years. The mortality rate from stroke in the United States also decreased by more than 5 percent per year from 1970 to 1985 (down by 78 percent overall). Yet cardiovascular diseases are still the number-one cause of death and disability in Americans, and older persons are especially hard hit.

Previous studies using a somewhat inaccurate statistical technique referred to as the "risk ratio" showed that lowering cholesterol levels in older persons may not be as beneficial as it is in younger adults. Many concurrent diseases can lower the blood cholesterol—especially in older people who are prone to other problems—and make "risk ratios" misleading in this population.

A more accurate way of measuring the harmful effects of elevated cholesterol in older people is the "attributable risk." In this approach we look at the difference in the rates of coronary events among older persons with elevated blood cholesterol and compare them with those who have desirable levels. A recent study involving over 356,000 adults of all ages demonstrated that the risk attributable to elevated "bad" LDL cholesterol levels does in fact increase with age. A follow-up study of more than 2,700 men 60 to 80 years old also showed that the risk of dying from CHD that can be attributed to elevated blood cholesterol increased by as much as 500 percent over those 20 years.

One source of error and underestimation of the risk of elevated cholesterol levels in this age group is that invariably we apply those cholesterol levels termed "desirable," "borderline high," or "high" for the younger population to older persons. This is erroneous, because for many healthy older persons, cholesterol levels may rise by approximately 10 mg/dl for every five years past age 60. What is an elevated level of cholesterol when you are young may be acceptable when you are older.

Statistical and technical miscalculations have diluted the data on the elderly and may have created the impression that elevated cholesterol levels are not as important in this age group. In fact, the opposite is true; cholesterol-lowering interventions could potentially prevent more death and disability from CHD per year among the elderly than among the middle-aged.

Which Older Persons with Abnormal Cholesterol Need Intervention?

Because coronary heart disease is more common in older persons (over 10 percent of this group) than in younger ones (1 percent), a higher number of older persons may benefit from risk reduction measures, including a decline in levels of blood cholesterol. Clearly, those who have other major risk factors should make every effort to modify or treat coexisting problems.

Nearly one-half of older persons take more than one prescription drug. Medications can affect appetite or cause nausea, fullness, early satiety, and various other gastrointestinal side effects. Many elderly people are "nutritionally disadvantaged" for a variety of reasons, including poverty, chronic illness, living alone and not cooking for themselves, depression, and poor appetite. For them, imposition of a rigid diet or the addition of another drug to lower their cholesterol levels is not justified.

People who are 60 to 65 years of age are expected to live an additional 20 years or more, so intervention in this group is certainly more reasonable than in those who are 75 to 85 years old.

Older Women and Cardiovascular Events

Coronary heart disease is not for men only. Over half a million women die every year in the United States from cardiovascular diseases, more than twice the rate for all forms of cancer combined. It is estimated that of the more than 500,000 deaths each year from heart attack alone, approximately 247,000 occur in women, many within the first few weeks after heart attack.

The risk of cardiovascular events in postmenopausal women increases dramatically. Nearly 50 percent of these women have "high" blood cholesterol levels (greater than 240 mg/dl). As noted earlier, almost 80 percent of women with coronary heart disease have low levels of the "good" HDL cholesterol. When smoking or high blood pressure is figured in, the risk of developing various cardiovascular events soars.

Numerous studies have convincingly shown that treatment with estrogen after menopause reduces the risk of a coronary event by about 50 percent. This beneficial effect is seen even among older women or those with abnormal cholesterol levels. Estrogen replacement therapy not only lowers the "bad" LDL and increases the "good" HDL, it may also improve the resistance of the inner wall of the arteries to injury and reduce the spasm of coronary arteries. An almost universal concern about estrogen replacement therapy is whether it increases the risk of developing breast or uterine cancer. Recent long-term data suggest that such a risk in women with no previous breast cancer (or no family history of breast cancer) is so small that it is dwarfed by the cardiovascular benefits and dramatic reductions in the risk of bone fractures, disabilities, and deaths attributable to osteoporosis.

Between the ages of thirty and seventy, high blood cholesterol is twice as common in African-American men as in white men, and for African-American women it is three times as common as for white women. More disturbing is the fact that *severe* hypertension affects five times as many African-American men as white men and seven times as many African-American women as white women. Thus, older African-Americans with hypertension and elevated blood cholesterol, especially when accompanied by a low level of HDL, are at extremely high risk for cardiovascular events and require more attention and effort to reduce their risk factors.

The rate of coronary heart disease in older women lags behind that of men by almost 10 years. Yet CHD is still the most common cause of death and disability in older women. A recent long-term study of 115,886 women who were between the ages of 30 to 55 at the beginning of the study showed that obesity and various risk factors associated with it accounted for 40 percent of cardiovascular events in women. In fact, in those with severe obesity, 70 percent of all cardiovascular events were attributable to obesity-related risk factors (such as severe abdominal obesity, hypertension, elevated "bad" LDL cholesterol and triglycerides, low levels of "good" HDL cholesterol, diabetes, enlargement and thickening of the wall of the heart, and insufficient exercise).

On the other hand, numerous studies have shown that slight-to-moderate obesity without the associated risk factors has no major impact on coronary arteries. This is especially true for older persons who have no obesity-related risk factors and for whom weight loss does not provide any cardiovascular benefit.

There is a prevailing myth that women tolerate heart attacks or coronary heart disease better than men do. This is simply not true, and such a mistaken notion has contributed to less intensive intervention and attention to risk modification in women. In one major study, the risk of dying within one year after a heart attack was 45 percent for women as compared to 10 percent for men. Numerous other studies have confirmed a poorer prognosis for women with CHD, especially African-American women. A more responsive approach to prevention and treatment of cardiovascular diseases in women is gaining recognition.

A Sensible Approach to Intervention in Older Persons

Older persons already have two CHD risk factors: (1) age itself and (2) being a man or a postmenopausal woman. Over 70 percent of older Americans have elevated levels of cholesterol, and nearly one-half have high blood pressure. A large number of them also have additional risk factors. Under these circumstances, there should be no complacency in considering intervention, provided that concerns about convenience, choice, flexibility, minimal side effects, and quality of life are incorporated into the program. Simplicity, ease of preparation, food preferences, and especially cost are crucial features of nutritional intervention in this population. Older persons who are highly motivated to improve their cholesterol levels (for both LDL and HDL) and who are good candidates should be given the opportunity to decrease their cardiovascular risk. For them, a flexible dietary program based on the CEF Index is a logical approach.

In older persons, intensive measures to quickly reduce various risk factors such as inactivity, high blood pressure, elevated blood sugar (diabetes), and obesity are counterproductive and likely to result in side effects or complications. However, a flexible dietary program based on the CEF Index, smoking cessation, and gradual reduction of other risk factors are all reasonable measures.

Avoid Smoking

Contrary to prevailing views that it takes one to two years for any cardiovascular benefit to accrue after quitting smoking, many beneficial changes do occur within two to three weeks. In a recent British study, 30 long-term smokers were evaluated two weeks before and two weeks after they stopped smoking. Significant reductions in blood fibrinogen (a potent clot producer) and blood viscosity (thickness), as well as a significant increase in "good" HDL cholesterol levels, were noted two weeks after smoking cessation. Since smoking also causes a significant increase in coronary artery spasm and constriction, quitting smoking reduces the risk of heart pain (angina) and heart attacks almost immediately.

The relation of cigarette smoking to death rates from all causes—cardiovascular events and cancers—was recently reported after a five-year follow-up of more than 7,000 men and women over age 65. In both sexes, the death rate from all causes among current smokers was twice that among older persons who had never smoked. The risk of dying from cardiovascular causes was also twice that for smokers as compared to those who never smoked, whereas 2.5 times as many current smokers died of cancer as those who never smoked. The good news is that in both men and women, former smokers had rates of cardiovascular mortality similar to those who had never smoked. These and other observations suggest that, especially in this population, we should be assertive in our stop-smoking efforts.

Adequate Exercise

Most older people who get little or no exercise would benefit from an age-appropriate program. A recent study involving 1,019 men and 1,273 women ages 50 to 89 showed that exercise at levels attainable by older adults significantly raises the levels of the "good" HDL cholesterol. However, the most important cardiovascular benefit of exercise in older persons may be the dramatic increase (140 percent) in blood levels of an anticlotting substance the body produces, plasminogen activator. This increase, along with other favorable changes, effectively reduces the risk of heart attack, sudden death, and stroke. What is surprising is that these favorable changes are not as dramatic in younger persons. Preliminary studies also suggest that regular exercise can reduce or even prevent the arterial stiffening that often occurs in older persons. Better cardiovascular, digestive, and musculoskeletal functioning and a better quality of life are other benefits of exercise.

Strengthening the Immune System

Considerable evidence indicates that aging is associated with changes in the immune system, especially regarding the white blood cells that fight infection. One mechanism by which omega-6 polyunsaturates from vegetable oils suppress the immune system may be related to changes in the function of T lymphocytes. It has been shown that vitamin E supplements of approximately 400 to 800 milligrams per day in healthy older persons improve various immune responses. Moderate doses of vitamin E also have a theoretical antioxidant effect, reducing the level of the "mean" oxidized LDL. For these reasons, it may be sensible to supplement an older person's diet with vitamin E, especially if he or she increases the intake of omega-6 PUFA (vegetable oils, margarines, etc.). Although the long-term benefits of vitamin E supplements are purely theoretical, at these moderate doses they do no harm.

Prolonging the life span beyond 85 or 90 years is very difficult to achieve. But we should certainly aim to improve quality of life, reduce infirmity or suffering, and allow older people to live better—if not longer—lives.

22

Abnormal Blood Lipids in Children and Adolescents

The recent concern about screening all children to detect elevated cholesterol levels has created a great deal of confusion and uncertainty among parents and health-care providers. Before we draw any conclusion about the "evils" of elevated cholesterol in this age group, we need to clarify several issues.

Measuring Lipid Levels in Children

For most children and adolescents, the desirable level of total blood cholesterol is about 170 mg/dl (± 30 mg/dl). Therefore, the actual *normal* level can range from 140 mg/dl to 200 mg/dl. The corresponding number for both the "bad" LDL cholesterol and triglycerides is 90 mg/dl (± 30 mg/dl). Levels greater than 200 mg/dl for total cholesterol and 120 mg/dl for LDL cholesterol and triglycerides are considered elevated. For the "good" HDL cholesterol, any value below 50 mg/dl is too low.

Measurements of blood cholesterol and lipoproteins in children are subject to the same drawbacks as those in adults (chapter 1). If anything, most of these factors affect random cholesterol measurements in children more than they do in adults. In fact, no child should ever be labeled with "abnormal" or "elevated" levels of cholesterol unless and until at least two fasting lipoprotein analyses are carried out over a period of several weeks. This will confirm that such an abnormality really exists. A random, single needle-stick cholesterol test during childhood or adolescence is useless and should not be used to diagnose or treat elevated cholesterol.

Consequences of Abnormal Blood Lipids in Children and Adolescents

In the United States, approximately 5 to 10 percent of children have elevated levels of cholesterol. The number of those with low levels of the "good" HDL cholesterol is not known. However, considering the pitfalls of cholesterol measurement, the prevalence of elevated blood cholesterol in children is actually closer to 5 percent. One-third of these children will go on to have "borderline high" blood cholesterol levels (200–240 mg/dl) as adults, and another one-third will have high levels (greater than 240 mg/dl). Among children and adolescents with "normal" cholesterol, nearly one out of five will have similar levels (greater than 200 mg/dl) as adults. Clearly, cholesterol levels in adults cannot be predicted with any accuracy on the basis of childhood data.

Let us now take the worst possible scenario and assume that about two-thirds, or 65 percent, of children with elevated cholesterol will become adults with elevated cholesterol. Only a small fraction of adults (about 2 percent) with elevated levels will experience coronary heart disease; the other 98 percent will not. Thus the overall number of adults who could be "saved" from developing CHD if we screened all children is infinitely small—on the order of one adult for every 3,000 screened children. This, of course, assumes that all children with elevated cholesterol are successfully treated and their blood cholesterol is kept at normal levels throughout their lives, which is nearly impossible.

Elaborate calculations show that 100 to 200 boys with elevated levels of cholesterol would need to follow a "cholesterol-lowering diet" for 50 years to prevent one premature death from CHD.

Since death rates from CHD for women under age 65 are much lower than those for men, the number of girls who would need to follow such a diet for 50 years to prevent one premature death from CHD is 300 to 600. This is hardly practical, reasonable, or justified.

Who Should Be Tested?

Considerable debate exists regarding universal screening of children for elevated cholesterol levels. Screening millions of children would be enormously expensive and could lead to labeling and stigmatizing many children without any benefit for most of them. The American Academy of Pediatrics Committee on Nutrition and the Expert Panel on Cholesterol in Children and Adolescents (National Cholesterol Education Program) have opposed routine screening during childhood.

As noted, recent data have consistently shown that most adults with documented coronary artery disease have low levels of the "good" HDL cholesterol and apoprotein A-1, which is the cardioprotective component of the HDL. What is not known is the relation between blood levels of these two important markers during childhood and the future development of coronary artery disease.

The reason children have various lipid disorders is genetic. Also, children share the same environment and dietary habits or life-styles of the people they live with. A recent study showed that if we tested only children who have at least one parent with total cholesterol above 200 mg/dl, we would have a 98 percent chance of detecting all children with elevated cholesterol. In other words, selective screening would miss only 2 percent of children with elevated levels of cholesterol.

At present, a sensible approach is to test children and adolescents who have a parent, grandparent, uncle, or aunt with CHD that was diagnosed before age 55. Children with parents or siblings who have abnormal blood lipids, and overweight or obese children, should also be tested. For most of those children and adolescents, obtaining the ratio of total cholesterol to HDL is a reasonable screening test, followed by full lipoprotein analysis on two occasions, before diagnosis or treatment. However, for children with a family member who developed CHD before the age of 55 but who shows normal lipoproteins, we should also test for apoproteins A and B as well as the "mean" lipoprotein (a).

Treatment of Children with Abnormal Blood Lipids

Children (and adults too) are not aware of their abnormal cholesterol. Unlike treating a sore throat or other infection, there is no tangible reward or prompt relief from symptoms when one embarks on a cholesterol-altering program. For this and a host of other reasons, long-term dietary intervention to alter cholesterol levels—especially in children—is a formidable task. It is absurd and cruel to try to convince children and adolescents that they should go on a restrictive low-fat, low-cholesterol diet for the rest of their lives just to reduce, by a few percentage points the risk of dying from a heart attack when they are 50 or 60 years old.

The psychosocial impact of labeling a child with a disease, the family hardship, or the adverse physical consequences (including growth retardation) may far outweigh the unproven and at best minimal benefits of restrictive diets in children. The concern over a perceived threat from elevated cholesterol also entangles parents and children in a never-ending struggle over what or how much the child should eat. This is a frustrating battle that parents usually lose. Self-discipline and long-term motivation are fragile qualities in children. The knowledge of elevated cholesterol has a far less powerful impact in "reforming" a child or adolescent than knowledge about the effects of smoking, alcohol, and drug abuse—areas where our time and effort might be more productive.

A few children (approximately 1 out of 500) who have a familial disorder that causes high cholesterol have a greatly increased risk of premature cardiovascular events. For them, early intervention is unquestionably necessary. These and other children or adolescents with markedly elevated "bad" LDL cholesterol and/or very low levels of "good" HDL cholesterol can best be managed on a flexible diet based on the CEF Index. In fact, such a flexible plan, with a total daily CEF Index of about +30, is healthful for the whole family. Young, middle-aged, and older people can all lead healthier lives by reducing the risk of cardiovascular disease. The CEF Index is a simple, satisfying point system to help everyone develop better eating habits.

Selected References*

Chapter 1

1. Report of the National Cholesterol Education Program Expert Panel on detection, evaluation, and treatment of high blood cholesterol in adults. 1988. *Arch. Intern. Med.* 148:36–69.

2. American Heart Association. *1992 Heart and stroke facts.* Dallas: American Heart Association.

3. Sempos, C., R. Fulwood, C. Haines, et al. 1989. The prevalence of high blood cholesterol levels among adults in the United States. *JAMA* 262:45–52.

4. Denke, M. A., and S. M. Grundy. 1990. Hypercholesterolemia in elderly persons: Resolving the treatment dilemma. *Ann. Intern. Med.* 112:780–92.

5. Vorster, H. H., A. J. Benade, H. C. Barnard, et al. 1992. Egg intake does not change plasma lipoprotein and coagulation profiles. *Am. J. Clin. Nutr.* 55:400–410.

6. McNamara, D. J., R. Kolb, T. S. Parker, et al. 1987. Heterogeneity of cholesterol homeostasis in man: Response to changes in dietary fat quality and cholesterol quantity. *J. Clin. Invest.* 79:1729–39.

7. Edington, J., G. Moira, R. Carter, et al. 1987. Effect of dietary cholesterol on plasma cholesterol concentration in subjects following reduced fat, high-fiber diet. *Brit. Med. J.* 294:333–36.

8. Grundy, S. M., D. S. Goodman, B. M. Rifkind, and J. I. Cleeman. 1989. The place of HDL in cholesterol management: A perspective from the National Cholesterol Education Program. *Arch. Intern. Med.* 149:505–10.

*Listed in the order in which they are referred to in text

9. Wilson, P. W. F., 1990. High-density lipoprotein, low-density lipoprotein, and coronary artery disease. *Amer. J. Cardiol.* 66:7A–10A.

10. Miller, M., L. Mead, P. O. Kwiterovich, and T. A. Pearson. 1990. Dyslipidemias with desirable plasma cholesterol levels and angiographically demonstrated coronary artery disease. *Am. J. Cardiol.* 65:1–5.

11. Romm, P. A., C. E. Green, K. Reagan, and C. E. Rackley. 1991. Relation of serum lipoprotein cholesterol levels to presence and severity of angiographic coronary artery disease. *Am. J. Cardiol.* 67:479–83.

12. Miller, M., A. Seidler, P. O. Kwiterovich, and T. A. Pearson. 1992. Long-term predictors of subsequent cardiovascular events with coronary artery disease and "desirable" levels of plasma total cholesterol. *Circulation* 86:1165–70.

13. Sacks, F. M. 1992. Desirable serum total cholesterol with low HDL cholesterol levels: An undesirable situation in coronary heart disease. *Circulation* 86:1341–43.

14. Mogadam, M., S. W. Ahmed, A. H. Mensch, and I. D. Godwin. 1990. Within-person fluctuations of serum cholesterol and lipoproteins. *Arch. Intern. Med.* 150:1645–48.

Chapter 2

1. Hopkins, P. N., and R. R. Williams. 1981. A survey of 246 suggested coronary risk factors. *Atherosclerosis* 40:1–52.

2. Ostlund, R. E., M. Staten, W. D. Kohot, J. Schultz, and M. Malley. 1990. The ratio of waist-to-hip circumference, plasma insulin level, and glucose intolerance as independent predictors of the HDL cholesterol level in older adults. *N. Eng. J. Med.* 322:229–34.

3. Gordon, D. J., and B. M. Rifkind. 1989. High-density lipoprotein—The clinical implications of recent studies. *N. Eng. J. Med.* 321:1311–16.

4. Buring, J. E., G. T. O'Connor, S. Z. Goldhaber, et al. 1992. Decreased HDL-2 and HDL-3 cholesterol, apo A-1 and apo A-2, and increased risk of myocardial infarction. *Circulation* 85:22–29.

5. Reinhart, R., K. Gani, M. R. Arndt, and S. K. Broste. 1990. Apolipoproteins A-1 and B as predictors of angiographically defined coronary artery disease. *Arch. Intern. Med.* 150:1629–33.

6. Lauer, M. S., K. M. Anderson, W. B. Kannel, and D. Levy. 1991. The

impact of obesity on left ventricular mass and geometry. *JAMA* 266:231–36.

7. Seed, M., F. Hoppichler, D. Reaveley, et al. 1990. Relation of serum lipoprotein (a) concentration and apolipoprotein (a) phenotype to coronary heart disease in patients with familial hypercholesterolemia. *N. Eng. J. Med.* 322:1494–99.

8. Scanu, A. M. 1992. Lipoprotein (a). A genetic risk factor for premature coronary heart disease. *JAMA* 267:3326–39.

9. Genest, J. J., S. S. Martin-Munley, and J. R. McNamara. 1992. Familial lipoprotein disorders in patients with premature coronary artery disease. *Circulation* 85:2025–33.

10. Austin, M. A., J. L. Breslow, C. H. Hennekens, J. E. Buring, W. C. Willett, and R. M. Kraus. 1988. Low-density lipoprotein subclass patterns and risk of myocardial infarction. *JAMA* 260:1917–21.

11. Badimon, J. J., L. Badimon, and V. Fuster. 1990. Regression of atherosclerotic lesions by high-density lipoprotein plasma fraction in the cholesterol-fed rabbit. *J. Clin. Invest.* 85:1234–41.

12. Brunzell, J. D., and M. A. Austin. 1989. Plasma triglyceride levels and coronary disease. *N. Eng. J. Med.* 320:1273–75.

13. Nestel, P. J. 1990. New lipoprotein profiles and coronary heart disease: Improving precision of risk. *Circulation* 82:649–51.

14. Davignon, J., R. E. Gregg, and C. F. Sing. 1988. Apolipoprotein E polymorphism and atherosclerosis. *Arteriosclerosis* 8:1–21.

15. Miettinen, T. A., and Y. A. Kesaniemi. 1989. Cholesterol absorption: Regulation of cholesterol synthesis and elimination and within-population variations of serum cholesterol levels. *Am. J. Clin. Nutr.* 49:629–35.

16. Muldoon, M. F., S. B. Manuck, and K. A. Mathews. 1990. Lowering cholesterol concentrations and mortality: A quantitative review of primary prevention trials. *Brit. Med. J.* 301:309–14.

17. Cunningham, M. J., and R. C. Pasternak. 1988. The role of viruses in the pathogenesis of atherosclerosis. *Circulation* 77:964–77.

18. Melnick, J. L., E. Adam, and M. E. DeBakey. 1990. Possible role of cytomegalovirus in atherogenesis. *JAMA* 263:2204–7.

19. Saikku, P., M. Leinonen, M. K. Mattila, et al. 1988. Serological evidence of an association of a novel chlamydia TWAR, with chronic coronary heart disease and acute myocardial infarction. *Lancet* 2:983–85.

20. Regnstrom, J., J. Nilsson, P. Tornvall, et al. 1992. Susceptibility to low-density lipoprotein oxidation and coronary atherosclerosis in man. *Lancet* 339:1183–86.

21. Manson, J. E., H. Tosteson, P. M. Ridker, et al. 1992. The primary prevention of myocardial infarction. *N. Eng. J. Med.* 326:1406–16.

22. Lowe, G. D. O. 1992. Blood viscosity, lipoproteins and cardiovascular risk. *Circulation* 85:2329–31.

23. Bairati, I., L. Roy, and F. Meyer. 1992. Double-blind, randomized, controlled trial of fish-oil supplements in prevention of recurrence of stenosis after coronary angioplasty. *Circulation* 85:950–56.

24. Stampfer, M. J., M. R. Malinow, W. C. Willett, et al. 1992. A prospective study of plasma homocyst(e)ine and risk of myocardial infarction in U.S. physicians. *JAMA* 268:879–81.

25. Ubbink, J. B., W. J. Hayward Vermaak, A. van der Merwe, and P. J. Becker. 1993. Vitamin B-12, vitamin B-6, and folate nutritional status in men with hyperhomocysteinemia. *Am. J. Clin. Nutr.* 57:47–53.

26. Phillips, A., A. G. Shaper, and P. H. Whincup. 1989. Association between serum albumin and mortality from cardiovascular disease, cancer, and other causes. *Lancet* 2:1434–36.

27. Barker, D. J. P., P. D. Winter, C. Osmond, B. Margetts, and S. J. Simmonds. 1989. Weight in infancy and death from ischemic heart disease. *Lancet* 2:577–80.

28. Leaf, A. 1990. Cardiovascular effects of fish oils: Beyond the platelet. *Circulation* 82:624–28.

29. McLennan, P. L., M. Y. Abeywardena, and J. S. Charnock. 1988. Dietary fish oil prevents ventricular fibrillation following coronary artery occlusion and reperfusion. *Am. Heart. J.* 116:709–17.

30. Burr, M. L., A. M. Fehily, J. F. Gilbert, et al. 1989. Effects of changes in fat, fish, and fiber intakes on death and myocardial reinfarction: Diet and Reinfarction Trial (DART). *Lancet* 2:757–61.

31. Radack, K., C. Deck, and G. Huster. 1989. Dietary supplementation with low-dosage fish oils lowers fibrinogen levels: A randomized, double-blind controlled study. *Ann. Intern. Med.* 111:757–58.

32. P. L. McLennan, M. Y. Abeywardena, and J. S. Charnock. 1990. Reversal of the arrhythmogenic effects of long-term saturated fatty acid intake by dietary n-3 and n-6 polyunsaturated fatty acids. *Am. J. Clin. Nutr.* 51:53–58.

33. Reimersa, R. A., D. A. Wood, C. C. A. MacIntyre, et al. 1991. Risk of angina pectoris and plasma concentrations of vitamins A, C, and E, and carotene. *Lancet* 337:1–5.

34. Steinberg, D. 1992. Antioxidants in the prevention of human atherosclerosis. The National Heart, Lung, and Blood Institute Workshop. *Circulation* 85:2338–43.

35. Blair, S. N., H. W. Kohl III, R. S. Paffenbarger Jr., et al. 1989. Physical fitness and all-cause mortality: A prospective study of healthy men and women. *JAMA* 262:2395–2401.

36. Thompson, P. D., E. M. Cullinane, S. P. Sady, et al. 1991. High-density lipoprotein metabolism in endurance athletes and sedentary men. *Circulation* 84:140–52.

Chapter 3

1. American Heart Association. *1992 Heart and stroke facts.* Dallas: American Heart Association.

2. Wilson, P. W., J. C. Christiansen, K. M. Anderson, and W. B. Kannel. 1989. Impact of national guidelines for cholesterol risk factor screening. The Framingham Offspring Study. *JAMA* 262:41–44.

3. Miller, M., L. Mead, P. O. Kwiterovich, and T. A. Pearson. 1990. Dyslipidemias with desirable plasma cholesterol levels and angiographically demonstrated coronary artery disease. *Am. J. Cardiol.* 65:1–5.

4. Romm, P. A., C. E. Green, K. Reagan, and C. E. Rackley. 1991. Relation of serum lipoprotein cholesterol levels to presence and severity of angiographic coronary artery disease. *Am. J. Cardiol.* 67:479–83.

5. Reinhart, R., K. Gani, M. R. Arndt, and S. K. Broste. 1990. Apolipoproteins A-1 and B as predictors of angiographically defined coronary artery disease. *Arch. Intern. Med.* 150:1629–33.

6. Grundy, S. M., D. S. Goodman, B. M. Rifkind, and J. I. Cleeman. 1989. The place of HDL in cholesterol management: A perspective from the National Cholesterol Education Program. *Arch. Intern. Med.* 149:505–10.

7. Assman, G., and H. Schulte. 1992. Relation of high-density lipoprotein cholesterol and triglycerides to incidence of atherosclerotic coronary artery disease (the PROCAM experience). *Amer. J. Cardiol.* 70:733–37.

8. Scanu, A. M. 1992. Lipoprotein (a): A genetic risk factor for premature coronary heart disease. *JAMA* 267:3326–29.

9. Seed, M., F. Hoppichler, D. Reaveley, et al. 1990. Relation of serum lipoprotein (a) concentration and apolipoprotein (a) phenotype to coronary heart disease in patients with familial hypercholesterolemia. *N. Eng. J. Med.* 322:1494–99.

10. Buring, J. E., G. T. O'Connor, S. Z. Goldhaber, et al. 1992. Decreased HDL-2 and HDL-3 cholesterol, apo A-1 and apo A-2, and increased risk of myocardial infarction. *Circulation* 85:22–29.

11. Austin, M. A., J. L. Breslow, C. H. Hennekens, J. E. Buring, W. C. Willett, and R. M. Kraus. 1988. Low-density lipoprotein subclass patterns and risk of myocardial infarction. *JAMA* 260:1917–21.

12. Badimon, J. J., L. Badimon, and V. Fuster. 1990. Regression of atherosclerotic lesions by high-density lipoprotein plasma fraction in the cholesterol-fed rabbit. *J. Clin. Invest.* 85:1234–41.

13. Brunzell, J. D., and M. A. Austin. 1989. Plasma triglyceride levels and coronary disease. *N. Eng. J. Med.* 320:1273–75.

14. Nestel, P. J. 1990. New lipoprotein profiles and coronary heart disease: Improving precision of risk. *Circulation* 82:649–51.

15. Davignon, J., R. E. Gregg, and C. F. Sing. 1988. Apolipoprotein E polymorphism and atherosclerosis. *Arteriosclerosis* 8:1–21.

16. Miettinen, T. A., and Y. A. Kesaniemi. 1989. Cholesterol absorption: Regulation of cholesterol synthesis and elimination and within-population variations of serum cholesterol levels. *Am. J. Clin. Nutr.* 49:629–35.

17. Manson, J. E., H. Tosteson, P. M. Ridker, et al. 1992. The primary prevention of myocardial infarction. *N. Eng. J. Med.* 326:1406–16.

18. Slyper, A. H. 1992. A fresh look at the atherogenic remnant hypothesis. *Lancet* 340:289–91.

Chapter 4

1. Anderson, K. M., P. W. F. Wilson, P. M. Odell, and W. B. Kannel. 1991. An updated coronary risk profile: A statement for health professionals. *Circulation* 83:356–62.

2. Manson, J. E., H. Tosteson, P. M. Ridker, et al. 1992. The primary prevention of myocardial infarction. *N. Eng. J. Med.* 326:1406–16.

3. Buring, J. E., G. T. O'Connor, S. Z. Goldhaber, et al. 1992. Decreased HDL-2 and HDL-3 cholesterol, apo A-1 and apo A-2, and increased risk of myocardial infarction. *Circulation* 85:22–29.

4. Genest, J. J., S. S. Martin-Munley, M. T. McNamara, et al. 1992. Familial lipoprotein disorders in patients with premature coronary artery disease. *Circulation* 85:2025–33.

Chapter 5

1. American Heart Association. *1992 Heart and stroke facts.* Dallas: American Heart Association.

2. Muldoon, M. F., S. B. Manuck, and K. A. Mathews. 1990. Lowering cholesterol concentrations and mortality: A quantitative review of primary prevention trials. *Brit. Med. J.* 301:309–14.

3. Sylkowski, P. A., W. B. Kannel, and R. B. D'Agostino. 1990. Changes in risk factors and the decline in mortality from cardiovascular disease. The Framingham Heart Study. *N. Eng. J. Med.* 322:1635–41.

4. MRFIT Research Group. 1990. Mortality rates after 10.5 years for participants in the Multiple Risk Factor Intervention Trial: Findings related to a prior hypothesis of the trial. *JAMA* 263:1795–1801.

5. Pekkanen, J., S. Linn, G. Heiss, et al. 1990. Ten-year mortality from cardiovascular disease in relation to cholesterol level among men with and without preexisting cardiovascular disease. *N. Eng. J. Med.* 322:1700–7.

6. Wilson, P. W. F. 1990. High-density lipoprotein, low-density lipoprotein, and coronary artery disease. *Amer. J. Cardiol.* 66:7A–10A.

7. Miller, M., L. Mead, P. O. Kwiterovich, and T. A. Pearson. 1990. Dyslipidemias with desirable plasma cholesterol levels and angiographically demonstrated coronary artery disease. *Am. J. Cardiol.* 65:1–5.

8. Manninen, V., P. Koshinen, M. Mantazzi, et al. 1990. Predictive value for coronary heart disease of baseline high-density and low-density lipoprotein cholesterol among Fredrickson type IIA subjects in Helsinki Heart Study. *Am. J. Cardiol.* 66:24A–27A.

9. Rossouw, J. E., B. Lewis, and B. M. Rifkind. 1990. The value of lowering cholesterol after myocardial infarction. *N. Eng. J. Med.* 323:1112–19.

Chapter 6

1. Vorster, H. H., A. J. Benade, H. C. Barnard, et al. 1992. Egg intake does not change plasma lipoprotein and coagulation profiles. *Am. J. Clin. Nutr.* 55:400–410.

2. McNamara, D. J., R. Kolb, T. S. Parker, et al. 1987. Heterogeneity of

cholesterol homeostasis in man: Response to changes in dietary fat quality and cholesterol quantity. *J. Clin. Invest.* 79:1729–39.

3. Edington, J., G. Moira, R. Carter, et al. 1987. Effect of dietary cholesterol on plasma cholesterol concentration in subjects following reduced fat, high-fiber diet. *Brit. Med. J.* 294:333–36.

4. Davignon, J., R. E. Gregg, and C. F. Sing. 1988. Apolipoprotein E polymorphism and atherosclerosis. *Arteriosclerosis* 8:1–21.

5. Miettinen, T. A., and Y. A. Kesaniemi. 1989. Cholesterol absorption: Regulation of cholesterol synthesis and elimination and within-population variations of serum cholesterol levels. *Am. J. Clin. Nutr.* 49:629–35.

6. Kern, F. 1991. Normal plasma cholesterol in an 88-year-old man who eats 25 eggs a day—mechanism of adaptation. *N. Eng. J. Med.* 324:896–99.

7. Russel, D. W., M. S. Brown, and J. L. Goldstein. 1989. Different combinations of cysteine-rich repeats mediate binding of low-density lipoprotein receptors to two different proteins. *J. Biol. Chem.* 264:21682–88.

8. Soutar, A. K. 1992. Familial hypercholesterolemia and LDL receptor mutations. *J. Intern. Med.* 231:633–41.

9. Leighton, R. F., F. J. Repka, T. J. Birk, et al. 1990. The Toledo exercise and diet study: Results at 26 weeks. *Arch. Intern. Med.* 150:1016–20.

10. Mogadam, M., S. W. Ahmed, A. H. Mensch, and I. D. Godwin. 1990. Within-person fluctuations of serum cholesterol and lipoproteins. *Arch. Intern. Med.* 150:1645–48.

11. Manson, J. E., H. Tosteson, P. M. Ridker, et al. 1992. The primary prevention of myocardial infarction. *N. Eng. J. Med.* 326:1406–16.

12. Hopkins, P. N. 1992. Effects of dietary cholesterol on serum cholesterol: A meta-analysis and review. *Am. J. Clin. Nutr.* 55:1060–70.

Chapter 7

1. Grundy, S. M., and G. L. Vega. 1988. Plasma cholesterol responsiveness to saturated fatty acids. *Am. J. Clin. Nutr.* 47:822–24.

2. Woollett, L. A., D. K. Spady, and J. M. Dietschy. 1989. Mechanisms by which saturated triacylglycerols elevate the plasma low-density lipoprotein-cholesterol concentration in hamsters: Differential effects of fatty acid chain length. *J. Clin. Invest.* 89:119–28.

3. Bonanome, A., and S. M. Grundy. 1988. Effect of dietary stearic acid on plasma cholesterol and lipoprotein levels. *N. Eng. J. Med.*) 318:12444–48.

4. Thorogood, M., L. Roe, K. McPherson, and J. Mann. 1990. Dietary intake and plasma lipid levels: Lessons from a study of the diet of health-conscious groups. *Brit. Med. J.* 300:1297–1301.

Chapter 8

1. Simopoulos, A. P. 1991. Omega-3 fatty acids in health and disease, and in growth and development. *Amer. J. Clin. Nutr* 54:438–63.

2. Mensink, R. P., and M. B. Katan. 1989. Effect of a diet enriched with monounsaturated or polyunsaturated fatty acids on levels of low-density and high-density lipoprotein cholesterol in healthy women and men. *N. Eng. J. Med.* 321:436–41.

3. Report of the National Cholesterol Education Program Expert Panel on detection, evaluation, and treatment of high blood cholesterol in adults. 1988. *Arch. Intern. Med.* 148:36–39.

4. Reaven, P., S. Parthasarathy, B. J. Grasse, et al. 1991. Feasibility of using an oleate-rich diet to reduce the susceptibility of low-density lipoprotein to oxidative modification in humans. *Am. J. Clin. Nutr.* 54:701–6.

5. Constant, J. 1988. Nutritional management of diet-induced hyperlipidemia and atherosclerosis: Part VIII. *IM* 9:124–29.

6. Mensink, R. P., and M. B. Katan. 1990. Effect of dietary trans fatty acids on high-density and low-density lipoprotein cholesterol levels in healthy subjects. *N. Eng. J. Med.* 323:439–45.

7. Troisi, R., W. C. Willett, and S. T. Weiss. 1992. Trans-fatty acid intake in relation to lipid concentrations in adult men. *Amer. J. Clin. Nutr.* 56:1019–24.

8. Bennett, M., R. Uauy, and S. M. Grundy. 1987. Dietary fatty acid effects in T-cell-mediated immunity in mice infected with mycoplasma pulmonis or given carcinogens by injection. *Am. J. Path.* 126:103–13.

9. Mead, C. J., and J. Mertin. 1988. Fatty acids and immunity. *Adv. Lipid. Res.* 16:127–65.

10. Kinsella, J. E., B. Lokesh, S. Broughton, and J. Whelan. 1990. Dietary polyunsaturated fatty acids and eicosanoids: Potential effects on the modulation of inflammatory and immune cells. An overview. *Nutrition* 6:24–44.

11. Mogadam, M. 1988. Cancer and nutritional misconceptions: A perspective. *Am. J. Gastro.* 83:1346–51.

12. Birt, D. F. 1987. Fat and calorie effects on carcinogenesis at sites other than mammary gland. *Am. J. Clin. Nutr.* 45:203–9.

13. Cleland, L. G., M. J. James, M. A. Neumann, M. D'Angelo, and R. A. Gibson. 1992. Linoleate inhibits EPA incorporation from dietary fish-oil supplements in human subjects. *Am. J. Clin. Nutr.* 55:395–99.

14. Wahlqvist, M. L., C. S. Lo, and K. A. Myers. 1989. Fish intake and arterial wall characteristics in healthy people and diabetic patients. *Lancet* 2:944–46.

15. Kromhout, D., E. B. Bosschieter, and C. de L. Coulander. 1985. The inverse relation between fish consumption and 20-year mortality from coronary heart disease. *N. Eng. J. Med.* 312:1205–9.

16. Leaf, A. 1990. Cardiovascular effects of fish oils: Beyond the platelet. *Circulation* 82:624–28.

17. Bonaa, K. H., K. S. Bjerve, and A. Nordoy. 1992. Habitual fish consumption, plasma phospholipid fatty acids, and serum lipids: The Tromso Study. *Am. J. Clin. Nutr.* 55:1126–34.

18. Burr, M. L., A. M. Fehily, J. F. Gilbert, et al. 1989. Effects of changes in fat, fish, and fiber intakes on death and myocardial reinfarction: Diet and Reinfarction Trial (DART). *Lancet* 2:757–61.

19. Radack, K., C. Deck, and G. Huster. Dietary supplementation with low-dosage fish oils lowers fibrinogen levels: A randomized, double-blind controlled study. *Ann. Intern. Med.* 111:757–58.

20. McLennan, P. L., M. Y. Abeywardena, and J. S. Charnock. 1990. Reversal of the arrhythmogenic effects of long-term saturated fatty acid intake by dietary n-3 and n-6 polyunsaturated fatty acids. *Am. J. Clin. Nutr.* 51:53–58.

21. Bonaa, K. H., K. S. Bjerve, B. Straume, I. T. Gram, and D. Thelle. 1990. Effects of eicosapentaenoic and docosahexaenoic acids on blood pressure in hypertension: A population-based intervention trial from the Tromso study. *N. Eng. J. Med.* 322:795–801.

22. Harris, W. S., D. W. Rothrock, A. Fanning, et al. 1990. Fish oils in hypertriglyceridemia: A dose-response study. *Am. J. Clin. Nutr.* 51:399–406.

23. Van Houwelingen, R., H. Zevenbergen, P. Groot, A. Kester, and

G. Hornstra. 1990. Dietary-fish effects on serum lipids and apolipoproteins. *Am. J. Clin. Nutr.* 51:393–98.

24. Weiner, B. H., I. S. Ockene, P. H. Levie, et al. 1985. Inhibition of atherosclerosis by cod-liver oil in a hyperlipidemic swine model. *N. Eng. J. Med.* 315:841–46.

25. Davis, H. R., R. T. Bridenstine, D. Vesselinovitch, and R. W. Wissler. 1987. Fish oil inhibits development of atherosclerosis in rhesus monkeys. *Arteriosclerosis* 7:441–49.

26. Fisher, M., P. H. Levine, B. Weiner, et al. 1990. Dietary n-3 fatty acid supplementation reduces superoxide production and chemiluminescence in a monocyte-enriched preparation of leukocytes. *Am. J. Clin. Nutr.* 51:804–8.

27. Fuster, V., L. Badimon, J. J. Badimon, and J. H. Chesebri. 1992. The pathogenesis of coronary artery disease and the acute coronary syndromes. *N. Eng. J. Med.* 326:242–50.

28. Childs, M. T., I. B. King, and R. H. Knopp. 1990. Divergent lipoprotein responses to fish oils with various ratios of eicosapentaenoic and docosahexaenoic acid. *Amer. J. Clin. Nutr.* 52:632–39.

29. Bairati, I., L. Roy, and F. Meyer. 1992. Double-blind, randomized controlled trial of fish-oil supplements in prevention of recurrence of stenosis after coronary angioplasty. *Circulation* 85:950–56.

30. Hearn, J. A., B. C. Donohue, H. Baalbaki, et al. 1992. Usefulness of serum lipoprotein (a) as a predictor of restenosis after percutaneous transluminal coronary angioplasty. *Am. J. Cardiol.* 69:736–39.

31. Steinberg, D. 1992. Antioxidants in the prevention of human atherosclerosis. The National Heart, Lung, and Blood Institute Workshop. *Circulation* 85:2338–43.

32. Scanu, A. M. 1992. Genetic basis and pathophysiological implications of high-plasma lipoprotein (a) levels. *J. Intern. Med.* 231:679–83.

Chapter 9

1. Thorogood, M., L. Roe, K. McPherson, and J. Mann. 1990. Dietary intake and plasma lipid levels: Lessons from a study of the diet of health-conscious groups. *Brit. Med. J.* 300:1297–301.

2. Mensink, R. P., and M. B. Katan. 1989. Effect of a diet enriched with monounsaturated or polyunsaturated fatty acids on levels of low-density

and high-density lipoprotein cholesterol in healthy women and men. *N. Eng. J. Med.* 321:436–41.

3. Keys, A., A. Menotti, M. J. Karvonen, et al. 1986. The diet and 15-year death rate in the seven-countries study. *Am. J. Epidemiol.* 124:903–15.

4. Grundy, S. M. 1986. Comparison of monounsaturated fatty acids and carbohydrates for lowering plasma cholesterol. *N. Eng. J. Med.* 314:745–8.

5. Sirtori, C. R., E. Tremoli, and E. Gatti, et al. Controlled evaluation of fat intake in the Mediterranean diet; comparative activities of olive oil and corn oil on plasma lipids and platelets in high-risk patients. *Am. J. Clin. Nutr.* 44:835–42.

6. Keys, A. 1987. Olive oil and coronary heart disease. *Lancet* 1:983–84.

7. Grundy, S. M. 1987. Monounsaturated fatty acids, plasma cholesterol, and coronary heart disease. *Am. J. Clin. Nutr.* 45:1168–75.

8. Baggio, G., A. Pagan, M. Muraca, et al. 1988. Olive-oil-enriched diet: Effect on serum lipoprotein levels and biliary cholesterol saturation. *Am. J. Clin. Nutr.* 47:960–64.

9. Ginsberg, H. N., S. L. Barr, A. Gilbert, et al. 1990. Reduction of plasma cholesterol levels in normal men on an American Heart Association step 1 diet or a step 1 diet with added monounsaturated fat. *N. Eng. J. Med.* 322:574–79.

10. Williams, P. T., S. P. Fortman, R. B. Terry, et al. 1987. Association of dietary fat, regional adiposity, and blood pressure on men. *JAMA* 257:3251–56.

11. Mensink, R. P., M. C. Janssen, and M. B. Katan. 1988. Effect on blood pressure of two diets differing in total fat but not in saturated and poly-unsaturated fatty acids in healthy volunteers. *Am. J. Clin. Nutr.* 47:976–80.

12. Mata, P., L. A. Alvarez-Sala, M. J. Rubio, et al. 1992. Effects of long-term monounsaturated- vs. polyunsaturated-enriched diet on lipoproteins in healthy men and women. *J. Clin. Nutr.* 55:848–50.

13. Fuster, V., L. Badimon, J. J. Badimon, and J. H. Chesebri. 1992. The pathogenesis of coronary artery disease and the acute coronary syndromes. *N. Eng. J. Med.* 326:242–50.

14. Mustard, J. F., M. A. Packham, and R. L. Kinlough-Rothbone. 1990. Platelets, blood flow, and the vessel wall. *Circulation* 81(suppl. I):I24–I27.

15. Reaven, P., S. Parthasarathy, B. J. Grasse, et al. 1991. Feasibility of using an oleate-rich diet to reduce the susceptibility of low-density lipoprotein to oxidative modification in humans. *Am. J. Clin. Nutr.* 54:701–706.

16. Parthasarathy, S., J. C. Khoo, E. Miller, et al. 1990. Low-density lipoprotein enriched in oleic acid is protected against oxidative modification: Implications for dietary prevention of atherosclerosis. *Proc. Natl. Acad. Sci. USA* 87:3894–98.

17. Calquhoun, D. M., D. Moores, S. M. Somerset, and J. A. Humphries. 1992. Comparison of the effects on lipoproteins and apolipoproteins of a diet high in monounsaturated fatty acids, enriched with avocado and a high carbohydrate diet. *Amer. J. Clin. Nutr.* 56:671–77.

Chapter 10

1. Anderson, J. W., N. Zettwoch, T. Feldman, J. Tietyen-Clark, P. Oeltgen, and C. W. Bishop. 1988. Cholesterol-lowering effects of psyllium hydrophilic mucilloid for hypercholesterolemic men. *Arch. Intern. Med.* 148:292–96.

2. Swain, J. F., I. L. Rouse, C. B. Curley, and F. M. Sacks. 1990. Comparison of the effects of oat bran and low-fiber wheat on serum lipoprotein levels and blood pressure. *N. Eng. J. Med.* 322:147–52.

3. Davidson, M. H., L. D. Dugan, J. H. Burns, et al. 1991. The hypocholesterolemic effects of beta-glucan in oatmeal and oat bran: A dose-controlled study. *JAMA* 265:1833–39.

4. Thorogood, M., L. Roe, K. McPherson, and J. Mann. 1990. Dietary intake and plasma lipid levels: Lessons from a study of the diet of health-conscious groups. *Brit. Med. J.* 300:1297–1301.

5. Ripsin, C. M., J. M. Keenan, D. R. Jacobs, et al. 1992. Oat products and lipid lowering: A meta-analysis. *JAMA* 267:3317–25.

6. Mogadam, M., S. W. Ahmed, A. H. Mensch, and I. D. Godwin. 1990. Within-person fluctuations of serum cholesterol and lipoproteins. *Arch. Intern. Med.* 150:1645–48.

Chapter 11

1. Intersalt Cooperative Research Group. 1988. Intersalt: An international study of electrolyte excretion and blood pressure. Results for 24-hour urinary sodium and potassium excretion. *Brit. Med. J.* 297:319–28.

2. Alderman, M. H., and B. Lamport. 1990. Moderate sodium restriction: Do the benefits justify the hazards? *Am. J. Hypert.* 3(6, part 1):499–504.

3. Ascherio, A., E. B. Rimm, E. L. Giovannucci, et al. 1992. A prospective study of nutritional factors and hypertension among U.S. men. *Circulation* 86:1475–84.

4. Cappuccio, F. P. 1992. The epidemiology of diet and blood pressure. *Circulation* 86:1651–53.

5. MacMahon, S., R. Peto, J. Cutler, et al. 1990. Blood pressure, stroke, and coronary heart disease. Part 1, Prolonged differences in blood pressure: Prospective observational studies corrected for regression dilution bias. *Lancet* 335:765–74.

6. American Heart Association. *1992 Heart and stroke facts.* Dallas: American Heart Association.

7. Schucker, B., J. T. Wittes, N. C. Santanello, et al. 1991. Change in cholesterol awareness and action. Results from National Physician and Public Surveys. *Arch. Intern. Med.* 151:666–73.

Chapter 12

1. Brinton, E. A., S. Eisenberg, and J. S. Breslow. 1990. A low-fat diet decreases high-density lipoprotein (HDL) cholesterol levels by decreasing apoprotein transport rates. *J. Clin. Invest.* 85:144–51.

2. Wood, P. D., M. L. Stefanick, P. T. Williams, and W. L. Haskell. 1991. The effects on plasma lipoproteins of a prudent weight-reducing diet, with or without exercise, in overweight men and women. *N. Eng. J. Med.* 325:461–6.

3. Lauer, M. S., K. M. Anderson, W. B. Kannel, and D. Levy. 1991. The impact of obesity on left ventricular mass and geometry. *JAMA* 266:231–36.

4. Buring, J. E., G. T. O'Connor, S. Z. Goldhaber, et al. 1992. Decreased HDL-2 and HDL-3 cholesterol, apo A-1 and apo A-2, and increased risk of myocardial infarction. *Circulation* 85:22–29.

5. Reimersa, R. A., D. A. Wood, C. C. A. MacIntyre, et al. 1991. Risk of angina pectoris and plasma concentrations of vitamin A, C, and E, and carotene. *Lancet* 337:1–5.

6. Gey, K. F., P. Puska, P. Jordan, and U.K. Moser. 1991. Inverse correlation between plasma vitamin E and mortality from ischemic heart disease in cross-cultural epidemiology. *Am. J. Clin. Nutr.* 53:3265–3345.

7. Steinberg, D. 1992. Antioxidants in the prevention of human athero-sclerosis. The National Heart, Lung, and Blood Institute Workshop. *Circulation* 85:2338–43.

Chapter 13

1. Reimersa, R. A., D. A. Wood, C. C. A. MacIntyre, et al. 1991. Risk of angina pectoris and plasma concentrations of vitamin A, C, and E, and carotene. *Lancet* 337:1–5.

2. Gey, K. F., P. Puska, P. Jordan, and U. K. Moser. 1991. Inverse correlation between plasma vitamin E and mortality from ischemic heart disease in cross-cultural epidemiology. *Am. J. Clin. Nutr.* 53:3265–3345.

3. Jialal, I., and S. M. Grundy. 1992. Effects of dietary supplementation with alpha-tocopherol on oxidative modification of low-density lipoprotein. *J. Lipid. Res.* 33:899–906.

4. Knopp, R. H., J. Ginsberg, J. J. Abers, et al. 1985. Contrasting effects of unmodified and time-release forms of niacin on lipoproteins in hyperlipidemic subjects: Clues to mechanism of action of niacin. *Metabolism* 34:642–50.

5. Wahlberg, G., G. Walldius, A. G. Olsson, and P. Kirstein. 1990. Effects of nicotinic acid on serum cholesterol concentrations of high-density lipoprotein subfractions HDL-2 and HDL-3 in hyperlipoproteinemia. *J. Intern. Med.* 228:151–57.

6. Lavie, C. J., L. Mailander, and R. V. Milani. 1992. Marked benefit with sustained-release niacin therapy in patients with "isolated" very low levels of high-density lipoprotein. *Am. J. Cardiol.* 69:1083–85.

7. Scanu, A. M. 1992. Lipoprotein (a): A genetic risk factor for premature coronary heart disease. *JAMA* 267:3326–29.

8. Steinberg, D. 1992. Antioxidants in the prevention of human athero-sclerosis. The National Heart, Lung, and Blood Institute Workshop. *Circulation* 85:2338–43.

9. Ascherio, A., E. B. Rimm, E. L. Giovannucci, et al. 1992. A prospective study of nutritional factors and hypertension among U.S. men. *Circulation* 86:1475–84.

10. Cappuccio, F. P. 1992. The epidemiology of diet and blood pressure. *Circulation* 86:1651–53.

11. Stampfer, M. J., M. R. Malinow, W. C. Willet, et al. 1992. A prospective

study of plasma homocyst(e)ine and risk of myocardial infarction in U.S. physicians. *JAMA* 268:877–81.

12. Ubbink, J. B., W. J. Hayward Vermaak, A. van der Merwe, and P. J. Becker. 1993. Vitamin B-12, vitamin B-6, and folate nutritional status in men with hyperhomocysteinemia. *Am. J. Clin. Nutr.* 57:47–53.

13. McCord, J. M. 1991. Is iron sufficiency a risk factor in ischemic heart disease? *Circulation* 83:1112–14.

14. Salonen, J. T., K. Nyyssonen, H. Korpela, et al. 1992. High stored iron levels are associated with excess risk of myocardial infarction in eastern Finnish men. *Circulation* 86:803–11.

15. Sullivan, J. L. 1992. Stored iron and ischemic heart disease: Empirical support for a new paradigm. *Circulation* 86:1036–37.

Chapter 14

1. Bak, A. A. A., and D. E. Grobbee. 1989. The effect on serum cholesterol levels of coffee brewed by filtering or boiling. *N. Eng. J. Med.* 321:1432–37.

2. Zock, P., M. B. Katan, M. P. Merkus, M. Van Dusseldorp, and J. L. Harryvan. 1990. Effect of lipid-rich fraction from boiled coffee on serum cholesterol. *Lancet* 335:1235–37.

3. Grobbee, D. E., E. B. Rimm, E. Giovannucci, G. Colditz, M. Stampfer, and W. Willett. 1990. Coffee, caffeine, and cardiovascular disease in men. *N. Eng. J. Med.* 323:1026–32.

4. Wilson, P. W. F., R. J. Garrison, W. B. Kannel, D. L. McGee, and W. P. Castelli. 1989. Is coffee consumption a contributor to cardiovascular disease? Insights from The Framingham Study. *Arch. Intern. Med.* 149: 1169–72.

5. Rosenberg, L., J. R. Palmer, J. P. Kelly, D. W. Kaufman, and S. Shapiro. 1988. Coffee drinking and non-fatal myocardial infarction in men under 55 years of age. *Am. J. Epidemiol.* 128:570–78.

6. Klatsky, A. L., G. D. Friedman, and M. A. Armstrong. 1990. Coffee use prior to myocardial infarction restudied: Heavier intake may increase the risk. *Am. J. Epidemiol.* 132:479–88.

7. Myers, M. G., and A. Basinski. 1992. Coffee and coronary heart disease. *Arch. Intern. Med.* 152:1767–72.

8. Myers, M. G. 1991. Caffeine and cardiac arrhythmias. *Ann. Intern. Med.* 114:147–50.

9. Rimm, E. B., E. L. Giovannucci, W. C. Willett, et al. 1991. Prospective study of alcohol consumption and risk of coronary disease in men. *Lancet* 338:464–68.

10. Puchois, P., N. Ghalim, and G. Zylberberg, et al. 1990. Effect of alcohol intake on human apolipoprotein A-1-containing lipoprotein subfractions. *Arch. Intern. Med.* 150:1638–41.

11. Shaper, A. G., A. M. Phillips, S. J. Pocock, and M. Walker. 1987. Alcohol and ischemic heart disease in middle-aged British men. *Brit. Med. J.* 294:733–37.

12. Regan, T. J. 1990. Alcohol and the cardiovascular system. *JAMA* 264:377–81.

13. Hillbom, M. 1987. What supports the role of alcohol as a risk factor for stroke? *Acta. Med. Scand. Suppl.* 717:93–106.

14. Stampfer, M. J., G. A. Colditz, W. C. Willett, F. E. Speizer, and C. H. Hennekens. 1988. A prospective study of moderate alcohol consumption and the risk of coronary disease and stroke in women. *N. Eng. J. Med.* 319:267–73.

15. Urbano-Marquez, A., R. Estruck, F. Navarro-Lopez, J. Grau, L. Mont, and E. Rubin. 1989. The effects of alcoholism on skeletal and cardiac muscle. *N. Eng. J. Med.* 320:409–15.

16. Beard, C. M., M. R. Griffin, K. P. Offord, and W. D. Edwards. 1986. Risk factors for sudden unexpected cardiac death in young women in Rochester, Minnesota, 1960 through 1974. *Mayo Clin. Proc.* 61:186–91.

17. Razay, G., K. W. Keaton, and C. H. Bolton, et al. 1992. Alcohol consumption and its relation to cardiovascular risk factors in British women. *Brit. Med. J.* 304:80–83.

18. Renaud, S., and M. De Lorgeril. 1992. Wine, alcohol, platelets, and the French paradox for coronary heart disease. *Lancet* 339:1523–26.

19. Sharp, D. 1993. Coronary disease: When wine is red. *Lancet* 341: 26–27.

Chapter 15

1. Grundy, S. M., D. S. Goodman, B. M. Rifkind, and J. I. Cleeman. 1989. The place of HDL in cholesterol management. A perspective from the National Cholesterol Education Program. *Arch. Intern. Med.* 149:505–10.

2. Wilson, P. W. F. 1990. High-density lipoprotein, low-density lipoprotein, and coronary artery disease. *Am. J. Cardiol.* 66:7A–10A.

3. Miller, M., L. Mead, P. O. Kwiterovich, and T. A. Pearson. 1990. Dyslipidemias with desirable plasma cholesterol levels and angiographically demonstrated coronary artery disease. *Am. J. Cardiol.* 65:1–5.

4. Gordon, D. J., and B. M. Rifkind. 1989. High-density lipoprotein—The clinical implications of recent studies. *N. Eng. J. Med.* 321:1311–16.

5. Brunzell, J. D., and M. A. Austin. 1989. Plasma triglyceride levels and coronary disease. *N. Eng. J. Med.* 320:1273–75.

6. Nestel, P. J. 1990. New lipoprotein profiles and coronary heart disease: Improving precision of risk. *Circulation* 82:649–51.

7. Leighton, R. F., F. J. Repka, T. J. Birk, et al. 1990. The Toledo exercise and diet study: Results at 26 weeks. *Arch. Intern. Med.* 150:1016–20.

8. Wood, P. D., M. L. Stefanick, P. T. Williams, and W. L. Haskell. 1991. The effects on plasma lipoproteins of a prudent weight-reducing diet, with or without exercise, in overweight men and women. *N. Eng. J. Med.* 325:461–66.

9. Cole, T. G., P. E. Bowen, D. Schmeisser, et al. 1992. Differential reduction of plasma cholesterol by the American Heart Association phase 3 diet in moderately hypercholesterolemic, premenopausal women with different body-mass indexes. *Am. J. Clin. Nutr.* 55:385–94.

10. Brown, G., J. J. Albers, L. D. Fisher, et al. 1990. Regression of coronary artery disease as a result of intensive lipid-lowering therapy in men with high levels of apolipoprotein B. *N. Eng. J. Med.* 323:1289–98.

11. Cobb, M. M., H. S. Teitelbaum, and J. L. Breslow. 1991. Lovastatin efficiency in reducing low-density lipoprotein cholesterol levels on high-fat versus low-fat diets. *JAMA* 265:997–1001.

12. Taylor, W. C., T. M. Pass, D. S. Shepard, and A. L. Komaroff. 1987. Cholesterol reduction and life expectancy: A model incorporating multiple risk factors. *Ann. Intern. Med.* 106:605–14.

13. Browner, W. S., J. Westenhouse, and J. A. Tice. 1991. What if Americans ate less fat? A quantitative estimate of the effect on mortality. *JAMA* 265:3285–91.

14. Grover, S. A., M. Abrahamowicz, L. Jeseph, et al. 1992. The benefits of treating hyperlipidemia to prevent coronary heart disease: Estimating changes in life expectancy and morbidity. *JAMA* 267:816–822.

15. Ornish, D., S. E. Brown, L. W. Scherwitz, et al. 1990. Can lifestyle

changes reverse coronary artery disease? The Lifestyle Heart Trial. *Lancet* 336:129–33.

16. Loscalzo, J. 1990. Regression of coronary atherosclerosis. *N. Eng. J. Med.* 323:1337–39.

17. Bradford, R. H., C. L. Shear, A. N. Chremos, et al. 1991. Expanded clinical evaluation of Lovastatin (EXCEL) study results. *Arch. Intern. Med.* 151:43–49.

18. The European Study Group. 1992. Efficacy and tolerability of simvastatin and pravastatin in patients with primary hypercholesterolemia: Multi-country comparative study. *Am. J. Cardiol.* 70:1281–86.

19. Thorogood, M., L. Roe, K. McPherson, and J. Mann. 1990. Dietary intake and plasma lipid levels: Lessons from a study of the diet of health-conscious groups. *Brit. Med. J.* 300:1297–1301.

20. Brinton, E. A., S. Eisenberg, and J. S. Breslow. 1990. A low-fat diet decreases high-density lipoprotein (HDL) cholesterol levels by decreasing apoprotein transport rates. *J. Clin. Invest.* 85:144–51.

21. Clevidence, B. A., J. T. Judd, A. Schatzkin, et al. 1992. Plasma lipid and lipoprotein concentrations of men consuming a low-fat, high-fiber diet. *Am. J. Clin. Nutr.* 55:689–94.

22. Parthasarathy, S., J. C. Khoo, E. Miller, et al. 1990. Low-density lipoprotein enriched in oleic acid is protected against oxidative modification: Implications for dietary prevention of atherosclerosis. *Proc. Natl. Acad. Sci. USA* 87:3894–98.

23. Enstrom, J. E. 1989. Health practices and cancer mortality among active California Mormons. *J. Natl. Cancer Inst.* 81:1807–14.

24. Henkin, Y., D. W. Garber, L. C. Osterlund, and B. E. Darnell. 1992. Saturated fats, cholesterol, and dietary compliance. *Arch. Intern. Med.* 152:1167–74.

25. Bonaa, K. H., K. S. Bjerve, and A. Nordoy. 1992. Habitual fish consumption, plasma phospholipid fatty acids, and serum lipids: The Tromso Study. *Am. J. Clin. Nutr.* 55:1126–34.

26. Hulley, S. B., J. M. B. Walsh, and T. B. Newman. 1992. Health policy on blood cholesterol: Time to change directions. *Circulation* 86:1026–29.

Chapter 16

Please refer to selected references listed for Chapters 5 through 13.

Chapter 17

1. Bonanome, A., and S. M. Grundy. 1988. Effect of dietary stearic acid on plasma cholesterol and lipoprotein levels. *N. Eng. J. Med.* 318:12444–48.

2. Childs, M. T., C. S. Dorsett, I. B. King, J. G. Ostrander, and W. Yamanaka. 1990. Effects of shellfish consumption on lipoproteins in normolipidemic men. *Am. J. Clin. Nutr.* 51:1020–27.

3. Van Vliet, T., and M. B. Katan. 1990. Lower ratio of n-3 to n-6 fatty acids in cultured than in wild fish. *Am. J. Clin. Nutr.* 51:1–2.

4. O'Dea, K., K. Traianedes, K. Chisholm, H. Leyden, and A. J. Sinclair. 1990. Cholesterol-lowering effect of a low-fat diet containing lean beef is reversed by the addition of beef fat. *Am. J. Clin. Nutr.* 52:491–94.

5. Simopoulos, A. P. 1991. Omega-3 fatty acids in health and disease, and in growth and development. *Amer. J. Clin. Nutr.* 54:438–63.

6. Steinberg, D. 1992. Antioxidants in the prevention of human atherosclerosis. The National Heart, Lung, and Blood Institute Workshop. *Circulation* 85:2338–43.

Chapter 20

1. Muldoon, M. F., S. B. Manuck, and K. A. Mathews. 1990. Lowering cholesterol concentrations and mortality: A quantitative review of primary prevention trials. *Brit. Med. J.* 301:309–14.

2. Taylor, W. C., T. M. Pass, D. S. Shepard, and A. L. Komaroff. 1987. Cholesterol reduction and life expectancy: A model incorporating multiple risk factors. *Ann. Intern. Med.* 106:605–14.

3. Browner, W. S., J. Westenhouse, and J. A. Tice. 1991. What if Americans ate less fat? A quantitative estimate of the effect on mortality. *JAMA* 265:3285–91.

4. Bret, A. S. 1989. Treating hypercholesterolemia: How should practicing physicians interpret the published data for patients. *N. Eng. J. Med.* 321:676–79.

5. Rossouw, J. E., B. Lewis, and B. M. Rifkind. 1990. The value of lowering cholesterol after myocardial infarction. *N. Eng. J. Med.* 323:1112–19.

6. Thorogood, M., L. Roe, K. McPherson, and J. Mann. 1990. Dietary intake and plasma lipid levels: Lessons from a study of the diet of health-conscious groups. *Brit. Med. J.* 300:1297–1301.

7. Brinton, E. A., S. Eisenberg, and J. L. Breslow. 1990. A low-fat diet decreases high-density lipoprotein (HDL) cholesterol levels by decreasing apoprotein transport rates. *J. Clin. Invest.* 85:144–51.

8. Simopoulos, A. P. 1991. Omega-3 fatty acids in health and disease, and in growth and development. *Am. J. Clin. Nutr.* 54:438–63.

9. Thompson, P. D., E. M. Cullinane, S. P. Sady, et al. 1991. High-density lipoprotein metabolism in endurance athletes and sedentary men. *Circulation* 84:140–52.

10. Blair, S. N., H. W. Kohl III, R. S. Paffenbarger Jr., et al. 1989. Physical fitness and all-cause mortality: A prospective study of healthy men and women. *JAMA* 262:2395–2401.

11. Hein, H. O., P. Suadicani, and F. Gyntelberg. 1992. Physical fitness or physical activity as a predictor of ischemic heart disease? A 17-year follow-up on the Copenhagen male study. *J. Intern. Med.* 232:471–79.

12. Sylkowski, P. A., W. B. Kannel, and R. B. D'Agostino. 1990. Changes in risk factors and the decline in mortality from cardiovascular disease. The Framingham Heart Study. *N. Eng. J. Med.* 322:1635–41.

13. Wennmalm, A., G. Benthin, E. F. Granstrom, et al. Relation between tobacco use and urinary excretion of thromboxane A2 and prostacyclin metabolites in young men. *Circulation* 83:1698–1704.

14. Manson, J. E., H. Tosteson, P. M. Ridker, et al. 1992. The primary prevention of myocardial infarction. *N. Eng. J. Med.* 326:1406–16.

15. Feher, M. D., M. W. Rampling, R. Robinson, et al. 1990. Acute changes in atherogenic and thrombogenic factors with cessation of smoking. *J. Royal Soc. Med.* 83:146–48.

16. LaCroix, A. Z., J. Lang, P. Scherr, et al. 1991. Smoking and mortality among older men and women in three communities. *N. Eng. J. Med.* 324:1619–25.

17. Wood, P. D., M. L. Stefanick, P. T. Williams, and W. L. Haskell. 1991. The effects on plasma lipoproteins of a prudent weight-reducing diet, with or without exercise, in overweight men and women. *N. Eng. J. Med.* 325:461–66.

18. Ruys, T., I. Sturgess, M. Shaikh, et al. 1991. Effects of exercise and fat ingestion on high-density lipoprotein production by peripheral tissues. *Lancet* 2:1119–22.

19. Rimm, E. B., E. L. Giovannucci, W. C. Willett, et al. 1991. Prospective

study of alcohol consumption and risk of coronary disease in men. *Lancet* 338:464–68.

20. Razay, G., K. W. Keaton, C. H. Bolton, et al. 1992. Alcohol consumption and its relation to cardiovascular risk factors in British women. *Brit. Med. J.* 304:80–83.

21. Mata, P., L. A. Alvarez-Sala, M. J. Rubio, et al. Effects of long-term monounsaturated- vs. polyunsaturated-enriched diet on lipoproteins in healthy men and women. *J. Clin. Nutr.* 55:848–50.

22. Steinberg, D. 1992. Antioxidants in the prevention of human atherosclerosis. National Heart, Lung, and Blood Institute Workshop. *Circulation* 85:2338–43.

Chapter 21

1. Spencer G. 1989. *Projections of the population of the United States by age, sex, and race: 1988 to 2080.* Washington, D.C.: U.S. Bureau of the Census. (Current population reports. Series P-25. No. 1018).

2. Fries, J. F. 1990. The sunny side of aging. *JAMA* 23:2354–55.

3. Denke, M. A., and S. M. Grundy. 1990. Hypercholesterolemia in elderly persons: Resolving the treatment dilemma. *Ann. Intern. Med.* 112:780–92.

4. Bonita, R., A. Stewart, and R. Beaglehole. 1990. International trends in stroke mortality: 1970–1985. *Stroke* 21:989–92.

5. Costs and effectiveness of cholesterol screening in the elderly. Congress of the United States. Washington, D. C.: Office of Technology Assessment. (Paper 3, April 1989).

6. Malenka, D. J., and J. A. Baron. 1988. Cholesterol and coronary heart disease: The importance of patient-specific attributable risk. *Arch. Intern. Med.* 148:2247–52.

7. Rubin, S. M., S. Sidney, D. M. Black, et al. 1990. High blood cholesterol in elderly men and the excess risk for coronary heart disease. *Ann. Intern. Med.* 113:916–20.

8. Castelli, W. P., R. J. Garrison, P. W. Wilson, R. D. Abbott, S. Kalousdian, and W. B. Kannel. 1986. Incidence of coronary heart disease and lipoprotein cholesterol levels. The Framingham Study. *JAMA* 256:2835–38.

9. Muldoon, M. F., S. B. Manuck, and K. A. Mathews. 1990. Lowering cholesterol concentrations and mortality: A quantitative review of primary prevention trials. *Brit. Med. J.* 301:309–14.

10. Barrett-Connor, E., and T. L. Bush. 1991. Estrogen and coronary heart disease in women. *JAMA* 265:1861–67.

11. Goldman, L., and A. N. A. Tosteson. 1991. Uncertainty about postmenopausal estrogen: Time for action, not debate. *N. Eng. J. Med.* 325:800–802.

12. American Heart Association. *1992 Heart and stroke facts.* Dallas: American Heart Association.

13. Manson, J. E., G. A. Colditz, M. J. Stampfer, et al. 1990. A prospective study of obesity and risk of coronary heart disease in women. *N. Eng. J. Med.* 322:882–89.

14. Steingart, R. M., M. Packer, P. Hamm, et al. 1991. Sex differences in the management of coronary artery disease. *N. Eng. J. Med.* 325:226–30.

15. Feher, M. D., M. W. Rampling, R. Robinson, et al. 1990. Acute changes in atherogenic and thrombogenic factors with cessation of smoking. *J. Royal. Soci. Med.* 83:146–48.

16. LaCroix, A. Z., J. Lang, P. Scherr, et al. 1991. Smoking and mortality among older men and women in three communities. *N. Eng. J. Med.* 324:1619–25.

17. Reaven, P. D., J. C. McPhillips, E. L. Barrett-Connor, and M. H. Criqui. 1990. Leisure-time exercise and lipid and lipoprotein levels in an older population. *J. Am. Geriatr. Soci.* 38:847–54.

18. Stratton, J. R., W. L. Chandler, R. S. Schwartz, et al. 1991. Effects of physical conditioning on fibrinolytic variables and fibrinogen in young and old healthy adults. *Circulation* 83:1692–97.

19. Meydani, S. N., M. P. Barklund, S. Liu, et al. Vitamin E supplementation enhances cell-mediated immunity in healthy elderly subjects. *Am. J. Clin. Nutr.* 52:557–63.

Chapter 22

1. Lauer, R. M., and W. R. Clarke. 1990. Use of cholesterol measurements in childhood for the prediction of adult hypercholesterolemia. The Muscatine Study. *JAMA* 264:3034–38.

2. Newman, T. B., W. S. Browner, and S. B. Hulley. 1990. The case against childhood cholesterol screening. *JAMA* 264:3039–43.

3. National Cholesterol Education Program. 1991. *Report of the expert panel on blood cholesterol levels in children and adolescents.* Bethesda, Md.: National Heart, Lung, and Blood Institute.

4. Benuck, I., S. S. Gidding, M. Donovan, et al. 1992. Usefulness of parental serum total cholesterol levels in identifying children with hypercholesterolemia. *Am. J. Cardiol.* 69:713–17.

5. Genest, J. J., S. S. Martin-Munley, M. T. McNamara, et al. 1992. Familial lipoprotein disorders in patients with premature coronary artery disease. *Circulation* 85:2025–33.

6. Scanu, A. M. 1992. Lipoprotein (a): A genetic risk factor for premature coronary heart disease. *JAMA* 267:3326–29.

7. Hulley, S. B., J. M. B. Walsh, and T. B. Newman. 1992. Health policy on blood cholesterol: Time to change directions. *Circulation* 86:1026–29.

Glossary

Angioplasty. Removing some of the clogging and plaques from the arterial wall. This is usually done through special catheters inserted into the arteries. At times tiny balloons are passed through these catheters and placed within the narrow segments of the blood vessels. With repeated and gentle dilation of the balloons, some narrow segments can be expanded to allow adequate blood flow.

Apoproteins. Also called apolipoproteins (or apos). These important proteins "manage" or "drive" the lipoprotein cholesterol molecules. They direct where the cholesterol goes and what it does. The important cardioprotective apoproteins are A-1 and C-3, whereas apo (a) and apo B-100 damage the inner wall of the arteries.

Arteriosclerosis. Hardening (sclerosis), thickening, and loss of elasticity of the arteries. It is due to degenerative changes or calcium and fat deposits in the arterial wall. Thickening of the inner wall may cause narrowing or closing of the arteries. Many patients who suffer a stroke have arteriosclerosis, but those with heart attack have atherosclerosis (see below).

Atherogenic. Having the potential to cause the formation of atheroma (see below).

Atheroma. A plaque or deposit within the wall of the arteries. Atheroma is made of blood platelets, cholesterol and other fats, inflamed cells, white cells engorged with fat (foam cells), and injured or thickened muscle cells in the arterial wall. Atheromas are the principal cause of the narrowing of the arteries and poor circulation.

Atherosclerosis. A form of arteriosclerosis involving various arteries, especially coronary (heart) arteries, in which atheromas are formed and progressively clog up the arteries.

Cholesterol. One of many fatty substances in the blood and tissues of all animals.

Coronary heart disease (CHD). Various heart problems related to atherosclerosis and clogging of coronary arteries that supply the heart muscle with blood and oxygen. Often this is expressed as angina (chest pain indicating inadequate oxygen supply to the heart) or heart attack (sudden stoppage of blood circulation to a portion of the heart because of clogging of the arteries).

Endothelium. The thin inner lining of the arteries. Injury to the endothelium may be the most important factor in the process of coronary heart disease.

Enzymes. Important proteins within the human body that regulate or facilitate all body functions. They range from digestive enzymes to most delicate enzymes involved in the production of cholesterol, various brain neurotransmitters, and the growth of cancer cells.

Essential. When used in the context of the human body, implies that some substance must be provided through dietary intake, since the body cannot produce it. Some amino acids and fatty acids are essential for the functioning of the human body and must be supplied through the diet.

Fatty acids. These are the smaller components of the breakdown or digestion of various fats. There are several kinds of fatty acids: saturated, monounsaturated, and polyunsaturated.

Free radicals and **oxygen free radicals.** Every cell in the body is a nonstop giant factory where hundreds of biochemical reactions are constantly taking place. During these activities, unstable and toxic by-products called free radicals are produced, and they are highly damaging to the cells. Some have very unstable oxygen atoms (called oxygen free radicals). Normally, almost all of these unstable by-products are immediately neutralized within the cells by other chemicals, enzymes, and reactions. Excessive production (or reduced neutralization) of these free radicals may have important roles in certain cancers or damage to the heart muscle, lungs, and many other organs.

Hydrogenation. A process in which hydrogen is added to unsaturated fatty acids. This is done to convert a liquid fat (oil) into a solid state and improve its stability. Hydrogenation reduces the degree of unsaturation of fatty acids. It also produces some trans fatty acids and isomeric fatty acids (see **Isomer**). Many vegetable shortenings and margarines have both trans and isomeric fatty acids that contribute to their semisolid consistency.

Isomer. The look-alike of any chemical. It contains the same numbers of atoms of the same elements, but the structural arrangement and properties are different. For example, many drugs are isomers of inert substances.

Lipids. Various fatty substances, including those in the blood.

Lipoproteins. These are tiny pellets that contain various fats, or lipids, and proteins (hence, lipoproteins). Lipoproteins are nature's vehicles for transporting cholesterol throughout the body. Based on their physical compactness (density), lipoproteins are classified as very low, intermediate low, low, or high in density.

Macrophages. These are specialized white blood cells that often play the role of scavengers in various tissues. They gobble up bacteria, remnants of dead cells, and other debris, including LDL cholesterol.

Omega-3 and omega-6 fats (PUFA). Omega (or n) refers to the distance between the first unsaturated carbon and the left end of a PUFA chain. For example, if the first unsaturated carbon (or double bond) occurs 3 carbons from the left end of the PUFA molecule, it would be an omega-3, but if it occurs at carbon number 6, it is called an omega-6. Omega-3 is present in all seafood and some nuts (almonds, pistachios, pecans, and walnuts), as well as canola seed and soybean oil. Vegetable oils, margarines, and shortenings are mostly omega-6 fatty acids.

Oxidization. When a substance gives up electrons, it becomes oxidized. Certain chemicals or oxygen atoms take up electrons from other substances, such as LDL cholesterol. Because of their potential to oxidize certain substances within the body, these chemicals are called oxidants.

Oxygenation. The process of delivering oxygen to various tissues. Since oxygen is carried by red blood cells, uninterrupted circulation of the blood is essential for tissue oxygenation.

Psyllium (pronounced SILLY-um). A water-soluble fiber from the husk of a plant. Psyllium is used in cereals or as a supplement to provide additional fiber in the diet.

Receptor activity, receptor sites. To work properly in the body, many chemical and biochemical substances must enter various cells through specific receptors. If an adequate number of receptors are not available, or are already occupied by other substances, then receptor activity is low. For example, low receptor activity for LDL cholesterol prevents the LDL from entering the liver and other tissues for its disposal. Under these circumstances, LDL cholesterol cannot be cleared from the blood, and this will result in an elevation of the cholesterol level.

"Responder," "nonresponder." These terms are used in medicine to identify individuals who do or do not respond to a particular form of treatment or intervention. For example, many people are salt "nonresponders," meaning that no matter how much salt they eat, it does not affect their blood pressure.

Sterols. Chemicals found in foods from plant sources, sterols have distant similarities to cholesterol but may be helpful substances.

Thrombosis. Clotting of the blood inside an artery or vein. Thrombosis of a coronary artery chokes off the circulation, causing a heart attack. The same process in a cerebral artery results in stroke.

T lymphocytes (T cells). Special white blood cells that are enormously important in defending against bacterial and viral infections. When the number of T cells is abnormally low, immune defenses are broken down, making an individual very susceptible to certain infections and cancers.

Trans fatty acids. Substances produced during hydrogenation of vegetable oils, considered even more harmful than saturated fats by some researchers. These are isomers (mirror images) of polyunsaturated fats, but they have distinctly different biological effects.

List of Abbreviations

All abbreviations used in this book are recognized internationally and appear in both scientific and consumer-related materials.

CHD = Coronary Heart Disease

Fatty Acids

MUFA = Monounsaturated fatty acids

PUFA = Polyunsaturated fatty acids

SFA = Saturated fatty acids

Lipoprotein Cholesterol

HDL = High-density lipoprotein ("good" cholesterol carrier)

LDL = Low-density lipoprotein ("bad" cholesterol carrier)

IDL = Intermediate-density lipoprotein (another "bad" cholesterol carrier)

VLDL = Very-low-density lipoprotein (another "bad" cholesterol carrier)

Oxidized LDL = Oxidized low-density lipoprotein (the "mean" cholesterol)

Index

Food and Drug Administration (FDA),
41, 106
Framingham Heart Study, 22
Free radicals, 67, 70–71
Frozen foods, CEF Indexes of, 96–97
Fruits, 64–65
　CEF Indexes of, 95
　fiber in, 56–58
　in flexible diet, 109
　raising HDL by eating, 124

Genetic factors, 15
　LDL and, 30
Grains, 64–65
　CEF Indexes of, 94
　in flexible diet, 109

Hardee's restaurant chain, 102–3
Hardening of the arteries, *See*
　Atherosclerosis
Heart attack, 16, 36
　estimated risk of, 22–24
　incidence of, 25
　iron and, 71
　in older women, 133
　omega-3 polyunsaturates and, 46
　potassium and, 69
　trans fatty acids and, 40, 42
Heart rhythm irregularities, 48, 69, 76
Herbs, 113–14
　raising HDL by eating, 124
High blood pressure, 17
　in African-Americans, 133
　alcohol and, 76
　coffee and, 73
　in elderly, 135
　minerals and, 69
　monounsaturates and, 53
　omega-3 polyunsaturates and, 48
　salt and, 59–60
High-density lipoproteins (HDL), 7–12,
77–79
　alcohol and, 74–76
　carbohydrates and, 62, 64
　catecholamines and, 15
　in children, 138–40, 142
　dietary cholesterol and, 29
　dietary interventions to raise, 121,
124–27
　dietary restrictions and, 79–83
　drugs for altering, 129

in elderly, 133–36
fiber and, 57
low blood levels of, 18–21
omega-3 polyunsaturates and, 45
omega-6 polyunsaturates and, 39–40
phytoalexins and, 75
vitamins and, 67, 68
Holidays, 116
Homocyst(e)ine, 69
Hydrogenation, 40–44
Hypertension. *See* High blood pressure

Immune system
　aging and, 136–37
　iron deficiency and, 71
　omega-6 polyunsaturates and, 41–42
Insulin, 63
　alcohol and, 74, 75
Intermediate-density lipoproteins (IDL),
6–8
Iron, 70–71
Iron-deficiency anemia, 57
Ischemia, 16

Kentucky Fried Chicken, 104

Life expectancy, 25
Lignoceric acid, 41
Linoleic acid, 41–44
Lipoproteins, 6–9
　apoproteins and, 9–10
　analysis of, 11, 12
　See also High-density lipoproteins;
　　Low-density lipoproteins; Very-low-
　　density lipoproteins
Low-density lipoproteins (LDL), 7–12,
15, 77, 79
　carbohydrates and, 62
　in children, 138, 141
　dietary cholesterol and, 29–32
　dietary interventions to lower, 121–24
　dietary restrictions and, 79–83
　drugs for lowering, 129
　in elderly, 131, 133–35, 137
　elevated, 18–21
　fiber and, 57
　monounsaturates and, 53, 54
　omega-3 polyunsaturates and, 45, 49
　omega-6 polyunsaturates and, 39, 40
　oxygen-free radicals and, 70, 71
　polyphenols and, 75